DICTIONARY

of

VETERINARY SCIENCES

Published by:
Lotus Press

DICTIONARY
of
VETERINARY SCIENCES

Dr. V.K.Narula

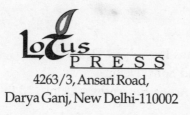
Lotus
PRESS
4263/3, Ansari Road,
Darya Ganj, New Delhi-110002

Lotus Press
4263/3, Ansari Road, Darya Ganj, New Delhi-110002.
Ph.: 32903912, 23280047, 9811594448
E-mail: lotus_press@sify.com ❑ www.lotuspress.co.in

Dictionary of Veterinary Sciences

ISBN: 81-8382-134-0

Published by: Lotus Press, New Delhi.
Printed by: Anand Sons, Delhi.
Laser Typeset by: Aruna Enterprises, Delhi-110 094

PREFACE

'Dictionary of Veterinary Sciences' has been compiled to include definitions of terms that may be encountered in various aspects of Veterinary Profession. An attempt has been made to present the terms in brief and avoiding more comprehensive description. The terms have been carefully selected from various Faculties in Veterinary Sciences which need to be referred and not merely a Veterinary Dictionary.

In the process of compilation and editing, our sincere effort was to make it a Reference book only. Effort has been carefully made to give clear and straight forward definitions with the aim of making terms understandable and perceivable by the readers.

The Dictionary of Veterinary Sciences is not an original work but a collection from various books on Veterinary and Allied Sciences. This will be of value for the students of Veterinary Sciences, especially useful for the Veterinarians working in the field practising in animal health regime, paravets providing first-aid to the animal populace in remote rural areas, as well as enlightened Poultry Farmers, Piggery Farmers, Stud owners and also the Pet Lovers. This can be of great help for the professionals working in the marketing of Veterinary Pharmaceuticals at various levels to enhance their technical skill for better communication with their prospectus.

Finally, the Editor expresses his sincere thanks to the publisher and printer for printing this book for the benefit of Veterinary Profession.

Inevitably, in a book of this nature, mistakes must have crept in and I would be grateful if readers would draw my attention so that the necessary corrections/ changes/editions can be made in the revised edition.

Dr. V.K.Narula

Terminology

In the beginning we may find Veterinary terms difficult to understand, pronounce, spell and remember. However, we must take an effort to learn because only then, we will be able to communicate fluently and effectively. This is not difficult, if we go about it in a methodical manner.

These are indeed derived form ancient languages. The key to understand them is the habit of analyzing i.e. breaking them into their component roots. For example, leuko means white, and cyto means a cell; thus leukocyte means a white cell (of the blood).

Terms fall into three categories. First, there are roots which refer to a part of the body, they are all nouns, secondly, there are roots which precede the nouns, i.e. they are used as prefixes, they usually qualify the noun and tell something about position, time, colour, fractions, multiples, speed, etc. Thirdly, there are roots which follow nouns, i.e. they are suffixes; they generally indicate a process, sensation, condition, disease, procedure, etc.

All terms contain a noun root. In addition, they have either a prefix, or a suffix or rarely both. The word leukocyte has a noun, viz. Cyto, and the prefix leuko. Endocarditis has all three types of roots : endo = inner (a prefix); cardia heart (a noun); it is = inflammation (a suffix). So endocarditis means inflammation of the inside of the heart.

You know that pneumo means lung and it means inflammation, you can build the word penumonitis and say inflammation of lungs.

Noun Roots

Adeno	=	gland	Logos	=	study
Algesia	=	pain	Myo	=	muscle
Angio	=	blood vessel	Nephro	=	kidney
Artho	=	joint	Neuro	=	nerve
Broncho	=	windpipe	Oma	=	tumour
Cardia	=	heart	Ophthalmos	=	eye
Cephalo	=	head	Osteo	=	bone
Cervico	=	rib	Patho	=	disease
Cyto	=	cell	Penia	=	deficiency
Derma	=	skin	Phagia	=	eating; appetite
Dypsia	=	thirst; drinking	Pharmaco	=	drug
Encephalo	=	brain	Pneumo	=	lung
Entero	=	intestine	Procto	=	anus
Gastro	=	stomach	Psycho	=	mind
Haemo	=	blood	Pyo	=	pus
Hepato	=	liver	Salpingo	=	uterine tube
Kerato	=	cornea	Stoma	=	mouth
Lipo	=	fat	Trophy	=	nourishment

Prefix Roots

A	=	absence of	Leuko	=	white
An	=	absence of	Macro	=	large
Ante	=	before	Mal	=	bad; poor
Anti	=	against	Mega	=	large; great

Auto	=	self		Mirco	=	small
Bi	=	self		Mono	=	one
Circum	=	two		Ortho	=	upright
Contra	=	opposite		Para	=	by the side
Di	=	two		Peri	=	around
Dys	=	painful		Poly	=	many
Ecto	=	outer		post	=	after
Endo	=	inner		Pre	=	before
Epi	=	above		Pseudo	=	false
Erythro	=	red		Retro	=	behind
Exo	=	outer		Semi	=	half
Hetero	=	different		Sub	=	below
Homo	=	same		Super	=	above
Hyper	=	excessive		Supra	=	above
Hypo	=	less		Syn	=	together
Idio	=	personal; private		Tachy	=	fast
Inter	=	between		Trans	=	across
Intra	=	within		Tri	=	three
				Uni	=	one

Suffix Roots

Aemia	=	presence in blood		Pathy	=	Disease
Algia	=	painful condition		Penia	=	Lack; deficiency

Asis	=	condition	Pepsia	=	digestion
Ectomy	=	removal	Phagia	=	eating
Emesis	=	vomitting	Philia	=	liking; attraction
Itis	=	inflammation	Phobia	=	fear
Lysis	=	dissolution	Plasty	=	repair
Oma	=	tumour	Rhoea	=	flowing
Osis	=	condition	Uria	=	presence in urine
Tomy	=	cutting			

Common Names

Animal	Male	Female	Young	Group	Giving Birth
Bear	Boar	Sow	Cub	Sleuth	Cubbing
Bird	Cock	Hen	Nesting	Flock	Hatching
Cat	Torn	Pussy/Queen	Kitten	Clowder	Queening
Cattle	Bull	Cow	Calf	Herd	Calving
Chicken	Rooster/ Cock	Hen/ Pullet	Chick	Flock	Hatching
Deer	Buck/Stag	Doe	Fawn	Herd	Calving
Dog	Dog	Bitch	Pup/ Puppy	Kennel	Whelping
Donkey	Jackass	Jennet	Colt	Herd	Foaling
Duck	Drake	Duck	Duckling	Flock	Hatching
Elephant	Bull	Cow	Calf	Herd	Calving
Fox	Reynard	Vixen	Cub	Earth	Pupping

Goat	Buck/ Billy	Nanny	Kid	Trip	Kidding
Hog	Boar	Sow/gilt	Piglet	Herd	Farrowing
Horse	Stallion/ Stud	Mare/Dam	Foal	Stable	Foaling
			Colt (M) *Filly (F)*		
Lion	Lion/ Tomi	Lioness	Cub	Pride	Whelping
Sheep	Ram	Ewe/Dam	Lamb	Flock	Lambing

COMPARISONS

Agile as a monkey

Bold as a lion

Cunning as a fox

Gentle as a lamb

Fast as a horse

Gaudy as a butterfly

Greedy as a dog

Light as feather

Hungry as a hawk

Obstinate as a mule

Merry as a cricket

Patient as an ox

Playful as a squirrel

Proud as peacock

Silly as a goose

Red as blood

Ugly as a toad

Watchful as a hawk

Slow as a snail

Sweet as honey

Tall as a giraffe

Timid as a hare

Warm as wool

A/a

- **Abattoir** A slaughter house.
- **Abaxial** Away from axis
- **Abdomen** Region of the body between thorax and pelvis containing the viscera other than heart and lungs (i.e. intestine, liver and kidneys, etc.). Also known as belly.
- **Abdominal cavity** This is largest cavity of the body which extends from the diaphragm to the pelvic inlet.
- **Aberration** A change from the normal. It is often used in reference to chromosomal abnormalities.
- **Abomasum** True stomach; the fourth compartment of stomach of cattle and other ruminants where actual digestion, similar to that in monogastric non-ruminant animals takes place.
- **Aboplety** Sudden marked loss of bodily function due to rupture or occlusion of a blood vessel.
- **Abortion** Expulsion of dead foetus prior to full gestation.

- **Abrasions** An injury in which alongwith the breaking of integument there is injury to the underlying tissue.
- **Abscess** A focal area of suppurative inflammation.
- **Absorbent** Able to take in or suck up.
- **Absorption** The passage of materials across a biological membrane.
- **Acanthosis** Thickening of epidermis prickle cell layer of skin.
- **Acaricide** A parasiticide effective against mites.
- **Acarology** The scientific study of mites and ticks.
- **Acetic acid** One of the volatile fatty acids with the formula CH_2COOH.
- **Acetonemia** see Ketosis.
- **Acetonuria** means that acetone is present in the urine.
- **Ache** To suffer a continuous pain.
- **Achorion** is a microscopic fungus causing honeycomb ringworm.

■ **Acid-Fast** Organisms are those which, when once stained with carbol-fuchsin dye, possess the power to retain their colour after immersion in strong acid solutions.

■ **Acidity** The quality of being acid or sour.

■ **Acidophilic** A bacterium or cell that has affinity for acid.

■ **Acidophilus** milk Fermented milk produced by inoculating Lactobacillus acidophilus in milk.

■ **Acidosis** A condition of reduced alkaline reserve of the blood.

■ **Aclalsia** Dilatation of oesophagus due to accumulation of food as a result of inability of the lower oesophageal sphincter to relax.

■ **Acne** Purulent inflammation of the hair follicle and sebaceous gland.

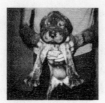

ACNE

■ **Acquire** obtain.

■ **Acquired immunity** The ability, obtained during the life of the individual, to produce specific antibodies.

■ **Acriflavine** A dye used as an antiseptic on skin and mucous membranes to disinfect contaminated wounds.

■ **Actinobacillosis** (Wooden tongue) It is a specific infectious disease caused by a bacterium—Actinobacillus lignieresi and is characterized by inflammation of the tongue also commonly affecting the pharyngeal lymphnodes and oesophageal groove.

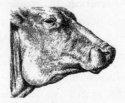

ACTINOBACILLOSIS

■ **Actinomycosis** ('Lumpy Jaw') in cattle is caused by Actinomyces bovis.

■ **Active** prompt, brisk.

■ **Active acquired immunity** That which the animal produces in his own body as a result of disease following by recovery or by vaccination.

■ **Acupuncture** The Chinese practice of piercing specific areas of the body along peripheral nerves with fine needles to relieve pain.

■ **Acute disease** Disease is called acute in contradistinction to 'chronic' when it appears rapidly and either causes death quickly.

■ **Acute** Having severe symptoms and a short course.

■ **Ad lib or ad libitum** Without constraint or limit, usually applied to feeding and watering.

■ **Adaptation** The adjustment of an animal to changing environmental conditions.

■ **Adapter** A device for connecting parts of an instrument or apparatus.

■ **Addict** A person exhibiting addiction.

■ **Addiction** Physiologic or psychologic dependence on some agent.

■ **Additive** An ingredient or a combination of ingredients added, usually in small quantities, to a food or feed for the improvement of shelf life or quality or nutritive value.

■ **Adenitis** means inflammation of a gland.

■ **Adeno** Gland

■ **Adenocarcinoma** Cancer of glandular tissue.

■ **Adenoma** A benign epithelial tumor in which the cells form recognizable glandular structures.

■ **Adenosine diphosphate (ADP)** The substance formed when ATP is split and energy is released.

■ **Adenotomy** Incision, or dissection of glands.

■ **Adenovirus** This is group of virus having DNA and causes infectious canine hepatitis.

■ **Adequacy** The state of being sufficient for a specific purpose.

■ **ADF (Acid detergent fiber)** Fiber extracted with acidic detergent in a technique employed to help appraise the quality of forages.

■ **Adhesion** The property of remaining in close proximity.

■ **Adhesions** Adhesions occur by the uniting or growing together of structures or organs which are normally separate and freely movable.

■ **Adhesive** Sticky

■ **Adipose** Of a fatty nature.

- **Adrenocorticotrophin Adipose tissue** A tissue comprising of cells containing fat and oil. It is found cheifly in major organs such as the kidneys and heart.
- **Adjacent** Near or next.
- **Adjuvant** Any substance used in conjunction with another to enhance its immune response to antigen.
- **Adrenal glands** A pair of endocrine glands situated immediately above the kidneys.
- **Adrenaline** A hormone which gets secreted by the medullas of the adrenal glands. It is also known as epinephrine.
- **Adrenocorticotrophin** Commonly abbreviated to A.C.T.H. It has been used in the treatment of acetonaemia in cattle, and is a naturally occurring hormone obtained from the anterior lobe of the pituitary gland.
- **Adsorb** To attract and retain other material on the surface.
- **Adulteration** Addition of an impurecheap, or unnecessary ingredient to a pure product.
- **Aerial part** The above-ground part of the plant.
- **Aerobe** is the name given to microorganisms which require oxygen, and consequently air, before they can grow and multiply.
- **Aerogen** A gas-producing bacterium.
- **Aerosol** A liquid agent or solution dispersed in air in the form of a fine mist.
- **Aesolute zero** The zero point on the absolute temperature scale-273.2°C.
- **Aesthesiology** Study of the organs of special senses
- **Aetiology** Possible cause of the abnormal state of health.
- **Affection** Tenderness.
- **Affinity** Attraction; a tendency to unite with another object.
- **Aflatoxicosis** Poisoning with aflatoxin.
- **Aflatoxin** Aflatoxins are common term used for a group of toxins and are produced by the fungi Aspergillus flavus and A. parasiticus under humid conditions.
- **Afterbirth** The membranes expelled from the uterus

following delivery of a foetus.

■ **Afterpains** are the rhythmic contractions of the uterus often assisted by the abdominal muscles (straining), resulting in the expulsion of the foetal membranes.

■ **Ag** Chemical symbol for Silver.

■ **Agalactia** Absence of milk from the udder.

■ **Agar** A complex polysaccharide derived from a marine alga and used as a solidifying agent in culture media.

■ **Age** The duration, or the measure of time of the existence of a person or object.

■ **Agent** Something capable of producing an effect.

■ **Agglomeration** Clustering, when milk particles collude amongst themselves and adhere to form clusters.

■ **Agglutination** Clumbing of bacteria erythrocytes or other cells due to agglutinins (Antibodies).

■ **Agmark** An acronym for agricultural marketing. A national insignia for quality and purity for agricultural and animal produce. Products bearing this insignia imply that they conform to certain grade specifications and standards laid down.

■ **Agony** Extreme suffering.

■ **Ailment** Any disease or affection of the body.

■ **Air** Atmospheric air contains by volume 20.96 per cent of oxygen, 78.09 per cent of nitrogen, 0.03 per cent of carbon dioxide, 0.94 per cent of argon, and traces of helium, hydrogen, ozone, neon, zenon, and krypton.

■ **Air Passages** These consist of the nasal cavity, pharynx, larynx, trachea and bronchi.

■ **Air sacs** In poultry, there are air sacs in the thoracic and abdominal cavity in bones etc. which help in respiration and also in flying.

■ **Al** Chemical symbol, aluminum.

■ **Alanine** One of the nonessential amino acids.

■ **Albinism** Individual having complete absence of melanin.

■ **Albumin** A class of water soluble proteins which coagulate on heating.

■ **Albuminuria** Presence of albumin in urine.

■ **Alcohol** A temperory stimulant but one which gives rise to later depression and is greatly inferior to those drugs mentioned under stimulants.

■ **Alcohol** test for milk A test whereas sour milk is coagulated.

■ **Aldosterone** Hormone which is secreted by the adrenal cortex and controls the excretion of salt and water through the kidneys.

■ **Aldrin** An insecticide. It is is a chlorinated naphthalene derivative used in agriculture against wireworms.

■ **Alfalfa** (lucerne) leaf meal The dried ground product consisting chiefly of leaves of alfalfa plant. Meal containing not less than 20 per cent crude protein and not more than 18 per cent of crude fibre.

■ **Algacide** Which kills algae is known as algacide.

■ **Algae** A group of photosynthetic eucaryotes; some are included in the Kingdom Protista and some in the Kingdom Plantae.

■ **Algin** A stabiliser which improves the whipping ability. It is particularly used in ice cream and chocolate milk.

■ **Alimentary canal** The gut—a tube leading from mouth to the anus. It includes mouth, oesophagus, stomach consisting of four compartments (rumen, reticulum, omasum and abomasum), small intestines, and large intestines.

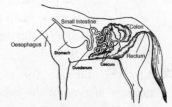

ALIMENTARY TRACT

■ **Alkali** is a substance which neutralises an acid to form a salt, and turns red litmus blue. Alkalies are generally the oxides, hydroxides, carbonates, or bicarbonates of metals.

■ **Alkali disease** Chronic selenium poisoning caused by consumption of seleniferous plants over a period of week or months.

■ **Alkalizer** An agent that causes alkali.

■ **Alkali therapy** Treatment with alkali.

■ **Alkali Neurea** An alkaline urea.

■ **Alkaline** Having more hydroxide ions(OH^-) than hydrogen ions (H^+); pH is >7.

■ **Alkaloids** Alkaloid means alkali-like containing amine groups and therefore may be viewed as ammonia derivatives.

■ **Alkalosis** Is a condition seen in ruminants due to excess production of Ammonia in rumen making the rumen liquor more alkaline.

■ **Allantois** It is a fetal membrane which develops from the hindgut.

■ **Allelomorphs, or alleles** Alternative forms of genes. Since genes occur in pairs in body cells, one gene of a pair may have one effect and another gene of that same pair (allele) may have a different effect on the same trait.

■ **Allergic dermatitis** is another name for eczema caused by an allergy.

■ **Allergy** Implied both increased and decreased sensitivity to foreign substances.

■ **Allethrin** An insecticide, C_{19}, H_{26}, O_2.

■ **Allograft** A graft between persons who are not identical twins.

■ **Allopathy** A system of therapeutics.

■ **Allotriophagia** Syn Pica

■ **Alloy** a solid mixture of two or more metals.

■ **Alopecia** Loss of hair due to metabolic deficiencies Alopecia may be the result of a hormonal imbalance.

■ **Alpha** First letter of the Greek alphabet 1.

■ **Altitude** Above sea level.

■ **Alum Aluminum** sulfate [$Al_2(SO_4)_3$].

■ **Alveolus** The tiny air sac in the lung of mammals and reptiles at the end of each bronchiole and is the site of exchange of respiratory gases.

■ **Amalgam** Alloy of two or more metals.

■ **Amaurosis** Partial or total loss of sight.

■ **Ambient** The prevailing or surrounding temperature.

■ **Ameba** A minute protozoon.

■ **Amebiasis** infection with amebas, especially with Entamoeba histolytica.

■ **Amenorrhoea** The absence or discontin uation or abnormal stoppage of the menstrual periods.

■ **Ametria** The congenital absence of the uterus.

■ **Amine** An organic compound containing nitrogen.

■ **Amino acid** Any one of a class of organic compounds which contain both amino (NH_2) and carboxyl (COOH) groups.

■ **Aminoglycoside** An antibiotic consisting of amino sugars and an aminocyclitol ring; for example, streptomycin.

■ **Aminophylline** A drug that relaxes smooth muscle and stimulates respiration. It is widely used to dilate the air passages in the treatment of asthma and emphysema.

■ **Amitosis** Direct cell division.

■ **Ammonia** is a pungent gas formed by heating a mixture of sal-ammoniac and quicklime.

■ **Ammonification** Removal of amino groups from amino acids to form ammonia.

■ **Ammonium** Hypothetical radical, NH_4.

■ **Amnion** A thin membrane forming a closed sac around the developing foetus. It contains amniotic fluid in which the foetus is immersed.

■ **Amoxycillin** This antibiotic resembles ampicillin, but is absorbed from the gut more quickly and to a greater extent.

■ **Ampere** Unit of electric current strength.

■ **Amphetamine** A sympathomimetic drug that has a very marked stimulant action on the central nervous system.

■ **Amphibia** The class of vertebrates that contains the frogs, toads, and salamanders etc.

■ **Amphistomes** are a type of fluke.

■ **Ampicillin** A semi—synthetic penicillin, active against both Gram-positive and Gram-negative bacteria. It is not resistant to penicillinase, but can be given by mouth.

■ **Ampoule** is a small glass container having one end drawn out into a point capable of being sealed as to preserve its contents sterile.

■ **Amylase** Any one of several enzymes which aid in the hydrolysis of starch maltose, for example, pancreatic amylase (amylopsin) and salivary amylase (ptyalin).

■ **Amylobarbitone** An intermediate-acting barbiturate, administered by mouth as a hypnotic in the treatment of insomnia or as a preoperative sedative.

■ **Amyloid** Homogenous translucent starch like substance.

■ **Amyloidosis** Deposition of amyloid in tissue.

■ **Anabolic agents** Refer to steroidal compounds that produce retention of nitrogen, potassium and phosphate.

■ **Anabolism** The conversion of simple substances into more complex substances by living cells.

■ **Anaemia** Qualitative or quantitative decrease in the amount of blood.

■ **Anaerobic** Living or functioning in the absence of air or molecular oxygen.

■ **Anaesthesia** Refers to a state of reversible unconsciousness which is induced by a general anaesthetic drug.

■ **Anal** Relating to the anus.

■ **Analgesics** Analgesics are drugs used for relief of mild and nonspecific pain.

■ **Analogous** Resembling or similar in some respects, as in function or appearance, but not in origin.

■ **Analysis** Separation into component parts or act of determining the component parts of a substance.

■ **Anaphase** The third stage of cell division, or mitosis, in which the doubled chromosome separates into identical chromatids.

■ **Anaphrodisiac** Refers to a drug that diminishes sexual desire.

■ **Anaphylaxia** Is an exaggerated reaction to a foreign protein which sometimes follows innoculation, stings etc.

■ **Anaplasmosis** The causal agent is anaplasma marginale. The disease starts with a high temperature of 105° to 107°F and after a day or two anaemia and icterus appear.

■ **Anatomy** Deals with the study of biological structures.

■ **Anchylostomiasis** A hookworm disease caused by _Anchylastoma sp._

■ **Andr(o)** Male; masculine.

■ **Androgens** Male hormones secreted by testis.

■ **Andrology** Study of male reproduction and its associated diseases.

■ **Anesthesiology** That branch of medicine, which studies anesthesia and anesthetics.

■ **Aneurin** is the vitamin B1, the anit-neuritic vitamin.

■ **Aneurysm** A localized dilatation of an artery, vein or a cardiac chamber.

■ **Angi(o)** Vessel (channel).

■ **Angina pectoris** A syndrome characterized by constricting parotysmal pain below the sternum most easily precipitated by exertion or excitement and caused by ischaemia of the heart muscle usually due to coronary artery disease.

■ **Angiography** A technique which enables the blood flow to and from a diseased organ to be visualised with the aid of single exposure or, preferably, serial radiography, after injection of a contrast medium.

■ **Angiology** Study of blood vascular and lymphatic systems.

■ **Angioplasty** Surgery of blood vessels.

■ **Angitis** or Angiits means inflammation of a vessel.

■ **Anhydrase** An enzyme that catalyzes the removal of water from a compound.

■ **Anhydrosis** Anhydrosis is a disease characterized by absence of sweating, occurring mainly in horses, and less commonly in cattle.

■ **Anhydrous** Containing no water.

■ **Animal** Any living organism of the kingdom Animalia, characterized by an inability to manufacture its own food.

■ **Animal drugs** Extracts or whole organs of animals employed therapeutically in the treatment of disease.

■ **Animal Husbandry** A branch of Veterinary Science

which deals with Livestock management, production and breeding.

■ **Animal protein factor (APF)** A growth factor (Vitamin B_{12}) present in animal feeds found absolutely essential for poultry and swine growth.

■ **Anisocytosis** Variation in size of erythrocytes.

■ **Ankylosis** A condition of a joint in which the movement is restricted by fibrous bands, by malformation by union of bones.

■ **Anode** The positive electrode or pole to which negative ions are attracted.

■ **Anodyne** Refers to a soothing medicine that relieves pain.

■ **Anoestrus** is the state in the female when no estrus or 'season' is exhibited. It is a state of sexual inactivity.

■ **Anomaly** Developmental defect affecting an organ or part of body.

■ **Anophagia or aphagia** Increased food intake.

■ **Anorectic drugs** Refer to drugs that depress the appetite and are used an aid to weight reduction.

■ **Anorexia** Complete absence of appetite.

■ **Anoscopy** Examination of the anal canal with an anoscope.

■ **Anoxia** Deficiency of oxygen.

■ **Antacids** A group of drugs widely used in human medicine to counteract the gastric hyperacidity of "nervous indigestion."

■ **Antagonist drug** A drug that counteracts or prevents the action of another drug or endogenous body chemical.

■ **Antemetic drugs** Drugs used for controlling vomition.

▣ **Ante-natal** Infection Infection which may occur before birth.

■ **Ante-partum** Paralysis common condition hindquarters of the pregnant animal suddenly become paralysed before parturition.

■ **Anterior** The front or forward part of the body.

■ **Anterior** Directed toward the front.

■ **Anteroposterior** Directed from the front toward the back.

■ **Anthelmintics Drugs** which destroy or expel helminthic parasites from the body e.g. Piperazine, Albomar etc.

■ **Anthracosis** Deposition of carbon in the lungs.

■ **Anthrax** Anthrax is a peracute disease characterized by septicaemia and sudden death with the exudation of tarry blood from the body orifices.

■ **Ante** Before.

■ **Anti** against.

■ **Antianginal drug** Refers to a drug which is used to relieve the pain and reduce the frequency and severity of attacks of angina pectoris.

■ **Antibacterial** Destroying or suppressing growth or reproduction of bacteria.

■ **Antibiotic** It is defined as a compound produced by a microorganism or a plant, or a close chemical derivative of such a compound that is toxic to microorganisms.

■ **Antibiotic resistant** Microorganisms that continue to grow and reproduce although exposed to an **antibiotic** are designated as **antibiotic** resistant.

■ **Antibody** Specific, protective substance produced by the body in defence against antigen (disease causing organism or foreign protein) and provides immunity against diseases by reacting with the antigen.

■ **Anticestodal Drugs** used to kill the tapeworm *in situ* or expels the living tapeworm.

■ **Anticoagulants** A variety of chemicals used to prevent coagulation of blood.

■ **Anticonvulsant drug** Refers to a drug that is able to prevent epileptic and related types of convulsion.

■ **Antidepressant** Preventing or relieving depression.

■ **Antidiarrheal** Counteracting diarrhea.

■ **Antidotes** Substances used to neutralise the effects of poison.

■ **Antifungal** Destructive to a fungi supperssing to growth or reproduction of fungi.

■ **Antigens** Foreign substances, mainly proteins, that stimulate formation of specific antibodies when introduced into the bodies of animals.

■ **Antihistaminics Drugs** which neutralise the effects of histamine in excess in the tissue.

■ **Anti-inflammatory** Counteracting or suppressing the inflammation.

■ **Antimony** is a metallic element belonging to the class of heavy metals.

■ **Antinematodal Drug**s Drugs used to combat parasitism of animals affected by nematodes.

■ **Antioxidant** Substances having the property of protecting other substances from oxidation such as Vitamin E protects unsaturated fatty acids by oxidising themselves.

■ **Antiperistalsis** is a term used to **indicate** a reverse action of the movements of the stomach or the intestines.

■ **Antipyretics** are drugs used to reduce temperature during fevers.

■ **Antirheumatic** Relieving or preventing rheumatism.

■ **Antiseptic** Substance which does not kill microorganisms but inhibits their multiplication or rate of growth.

■ **Antiserum** Serum for the use against a specific condition is produced by inoculating a susceptible animal with a sublethal dose of causal agent or antigen and gradually increasing the dose until a very large amounts are administered.

■ **Antispasmodics** are remedies which diminish spasm or 'cramp'.

■ **Antisterility** factor Vitamin E.

■ **Antitetanic** serum is a serum used against tetanus.

■ **Antitoxin** A specific antibody produced by the body in response to a bacterial exotoxin or its toxoid.

■ **Antitussive** A drug such as dextromethorphan or pholcodine that suppresses coughing, possibly by reducing the activity of the cough centre in the brain and by depressing respiration.

■ **Antiviral** Are agents used against virus.

■ **Antivitamins** Refers to substances that interfere with the function of vitamins or destroy them.

■ **Antizymatic action** Agents which prevent fermentation.

■ **Antrycide** A synthetic drug used in the control of trypanosomiasis.

■ **Anuria** Complete urinary failure.

■ **Anus** Posterior opening of the alimentary canal.

■ **Anxiety** Feeling of apprehension, uncertainty and fear without apparent stimulus.

■ **Aorta** is the principal artery of the body.

■ **Apathy** or depression Coma in which the animal is unconscious and cannot be roused.

■ **APC** Abbreviation for acetylsalicylic acid, acetophenetidin, and caffeine, used as an analgesic or antipyretic.

■ **Aphagosis** Inability to eat.

■ **Aphrodiasic** Refers to a drug that is able to stimulate sexual desire from aphrodite, the goddess of love.

■ **Apnoea** means the stoppage of respiration.

■ **Apodal** Without feet.

■ **Apoplexy** Sudden marked loss of bodily function due to rupture or occlusion of a blood vessel.

■ **Aposia** Absence of feeling of thirst.

■ **Apparent digestible energy (DE)** Absorbed energy, or apparent energy of digested food.

■ **Appendictis** Inflammation of appendix.

■ **Appetite** (Depraved appetite) Animal will eat rubbish such as cinders, coal, stones, soil, plaster, wire, old clothes, faeces etc.

■ **Appetite** Desire, chiefly desire for food.

■ **Aquatic** Growing in water.

■ **Aqueous humour** This is a clear fluid which occupies both anterior and posterior chambers of eyeball.

■ **Aqueous solutions** Solution or liquor is an aqueous solution of non-volatile medicinal drug of mineral or animal origin.

■ **Arachidonic Acid** A 20-carbon unsaturated fatty acid having four double bonds.

■ **Arachnoid** It is a very thin delicate membrane covers the brain and spinal cord.

■ **ARC** The Agricultural Research Council.

■ **Area under the curve** (AUC) Generally this term refers to the area under the curve which is relating plasma concentration of a drug to time after its administration.

■ **Areca-nut** is the seed of *Areca catechu*, the betel-nut tree.

■ **Argentum** The Latin word for silver.

■ **Arginine** One of the essential amino acids.

■ **Aromatics** include most of the essential oils of plants, such as cloves, turpentine, camphor, thymol and most are strong antiseptics.

■ **Arousal** A state of responsiveness to sensory stimulation.

■ **Arrhythmia** It is a rhythmical variation in heart rate.

■ **Arsenic** is a metal commonly used is the oxide, or arsemous acid.

■ **Arterial   Thrombosis** Arteritis leading to thrombus formation.

■ **Arteries** With the exception of the pulmonary artery, which carries venous blood to the lungs, these carry oxygenated blood from heart to body.

■ **Arteriosclerosis** Means hardening of arteries.

■ **Arthritis** Inflammation of the synovial membrane and articular surfaces joints.

■ **Arthrology** Description of joints or study of joints.

■ **Arthropathy** (Osteo-arthritis) Non-inflamatory lesions of the joint cavities.

■ **Arthrotomy** Incision of a joint.

■ **Articular** Pertaining to a joint.

■ **Artificial insemination** Is the deposit of male reproductive cells (sperm cells) in the female reproductive tract by mechanical means rather than by direct service of a male.

■ **Artificial vagina** (AV) A device used for collection of semen; simulating vagina. It consists of a thick rubber barrel casing fitted with a detachable rubber liner. At one end is placed a glass recepticle to retain ejaculated semen. Space between the rubber barrel / casing and liner is filled with warm water.

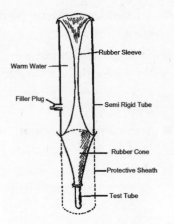

ARTIFICIAL VAGINA

■ **Ascariasis** Infestation by *Ascaris* nematode.

■ **Ascaridae** is the name of a class of worms belonging to the round variety.

■ **Ascites** Accumulation of dropsical or oedematous fluid in the abdominal cavity.

■ **Ascorbic acid** Vitamin C.

■ **Aseptic** When no pathogenic bacteria are present.

■ **Aseptic packaging** A process of filling sterilized liquid product, into a sterile package under sterile environment.

■ **Asexual** Having no sex.

■ **Asexual reproduction** Reproduction without opposite mating strains.

■ **Ash** The incombustible residue remaining after incineration at 600°C for several hours.

■ **Aspartic** acid One of the nonessential amino acids.

■ **Aspergillosis or Pneumomycosis** (Brooder pneumonia in poultry) caused by a fungus—*Aspergillus fumigatus*.

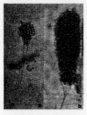

ASPERGILLUS

■ **Asphyxia** Difficulty in respiration or breathing due to insufficient oxygen supply to blood.

■ **Aspirated** Removal of light materials from heavier material by use of air.

■ **Aspirin (acetylsalicylic acid)** A widely used drug that relieves pain and also reduces inflammation and fever.

■ **Assay** A test to measure the amount of something.

■ **Assimilation** The process by which digested food is absorbed through the wall of the small intestine into the blood stream.

■ **Asthma** An allergic disorder of respiratory tract characterized by wheezing, difficulty in expiration and a feeling of constriction in chest.

■ **Astringent** Refers to a substance that brings about the denaturation of proteins so that they form a protective coagulated layer on mucous membranes or inflammed skin.

■ **Asuntal** An anti-tick organophosphorus compound.

■ **Asystole** means a failure of the heart to contract.

■ **Atavism** The reappearance of a character after it has not appeared for one or more generations.

■ **Ataxia** means the loss of the power of governing movements.

■ **Atelectasis** Failure of the alveoli to open and contain air i.e. collapsed alveoli.

■ **Atherosclerosis** Thickening of arteries par—ticularly elastic arteries in which there is deposition of soft mushy, glue like substance.

■ **Atlas** It is the first cervical vertbra.

■ **Atom** A particle or matter indivisible by chemical means. An atom consists of a dense inner core (the nucleus) and a much less dense outer domain of eletron in motion around the nucleus. Atoms are electrically neutral.

■ **Atomic number** The number of protons in the nucleus of an atom and also its positive charge.

■ **Atomic weight** The mass of an atom relative to other atoms; the atomic weight of any element is approximately equal to the total number of protons and neutrons in its nucleus.

■ **Atony** Flabbiness in muscles.

■ **Atrophic vaginitis** Inflammation of the vaginal mucosa secondary to thinning and decreased lubrication of the vaginal walls.

■ **Atrophy** Decrease in size of a cell, tissue, organ, or body part.

■ **Atropine** is the alkaloid contained in the leaves and root or the deadly nightshade (Atropa belladonna). Atropine is the antidote to morphine poisoning.

■ **Attenuation** Lessening of virulence of a microorganism.

■ **Audiovisual** The senses of both hearing and sight.

■ **Auditory** Pertaining to the ear or the sense of hearing.

■ **Auresky's** disease Syn pseudorabies

■ **Auricle (pinna)** Projecting outer portion of the ear.

■ **Auscultation** Direct listening to the sounds produced by organ movement is performed by placing the ear to the body surface over the organ with the help of stethoscope.

■ **Auto infection** Infection of one part of the body from another part.

■ **Autoclave** Equipment for sterilization by steam under pressure, usually operated at 15lb pressure and 121°C.

■ **Autogenous** Self-generated term used in association with vaccines, where the vaccine is prepared directly from the causal organism in a case of outbreak.

■ **Auto-Immune** Disease Is due to the defect or failure of body defence mechanisms in which antibodies become active against some of the host's own cells.

■ **Autolysis** Self digestion.

■ **Automatic** Spontaneous, done involuntarily.

■ **Autonomic nervous system** This is the visceral component of the nervous system. The nerve fibers are distributed to the viscera, blood vessels, glands and unstriped muscles.

■ **Autopsy** The examination of internal structure of the body performed after death. The term is used only in human beings.

■ **Autosomal genes** Genes located on any chromosome other than the sex chromosomes.

■ **Auto-trophic** Organisms which can use carbon dioxide as a sole source of carbon are called autotrophic.

■ **Autumn Fly** (Musca autumnalis) This is a non-biting fly which is a serious pest of grazing from live-stock.

■ **Avascular** Bloodless.

■ **Avermectins** Refer to a group of broad-spectrum antiparasitic drugs, both for ecto and endo parasites.

■ **Avian encephalomyelitis** A viral disease of poultry.

■ **Avian infectious encephal-omy-elitis** A disease of chicks under 6 weeks old.

■ **Avian infectious laryngotra-cheitis** of poultry is caused by a Herpes virus.

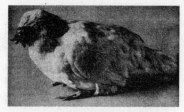

LARYNGOTRACHEITIS

■ **Avian leukosis** This is caused by Avian RNA tumour viruses.

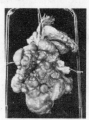

AVIAN LEUKOSIS

■ **Avian leukosis complex** A virus disease of birds charac-terized by a semi-neoplastic proliferation of leukocyte precursors (and at the same time erythrocytes also).

■ **Avian listeriosis** An infection disease of poultry, occuring as an epidermic among young stock. It is caused by *Listeria monocytogenes.*

■ **Avian** Of or pertaining to birds.

■ **Avian plague** or Fowl plague An avian influenza A virus.

■ **Avian tuberculosis** Disease of poultry due to the *Mycobacterium tuberculosis* (avian).

■ **Avidin** A protein in egg albumen which can combine with biotin to render the lat-ter unavailable to the animal.

■ **Avirulence** Lack of virulence.

■ **Avitaminosis** A diseased condition produced by a deficiency of a Vitamin in the food.

■ **Axial** Towards central line of the body

■ **Axis** It is the second cervical vertebra.

■ **Azoospermia** The absence of spermatozoa in the semen.

■ **Azoturia** Syn Myoglob-inuria, Monday morning disease, seen in horses. When suddenly put to exercise after a rest period of couple of days and fed over this period with diet rich in carbohy-drate.

❑

- **B. Cells** One of the two types of lymphocytes important in the provision of immunity, they respond to antigens.
- **b.i.d.** twice in a day
- **B.M.R.** Basal metabolic rate.
- **Ba** Chemical symbol, barium.
- **Babesiosis** Diseases caused by Babesia spp. characterized by fever and intravascular haemolysis causing a syndrome of anaemia, and haemoglobinuria.
- **Baby pig disease** Neonatal hypoglycaemia in piglets.
- **Bacillary Haemoglobinuria** Acute, highly fatal infection of cattle and sheep and is characterized clinically by a high fever, haemoglobinuria, jaundice, and presence of necrotic infarcts in the liver.
- **Bacillary White Diarrhoea** Disease of chickens caused by *Salmonella, pullorum.*
- **Bacillus** A genus of bacterial(family bacillaceae), including gram-positive, spore forming bacteria.
- **Bacillus** or **Bacilli** Bacteria which are rod shaped are called bacilli.
- **Bacillosis** Infection with bacilli.
- **Backbone** The Vertebral column.
- **Backcross** Mating a crossbred cow back to a bull from one of its two parental breeds.
- **Bacon** The cured and smoked fat and lean meat from the side of the pig, after the spareribs have been removed.
- **Bacteraemia** It is a general term, which denotes the presence of bacteria in the blood-vascular system.
- **Bacteria** Microorganisms according to peculiarities in shape and in group formation, certain names are applied.
- **Bactericidal** The agent which kills bacteria.
- **Bacteriocin** Toxic protein produced by bacteria that kills other bacteria.
- **Bacteriology** It is the branch of biology which deals with the study of bacteria.

- **Bacteriophage** A virus which attacks and destroys bacteria.

- **Bacteriostatic** Substances which control the growth of bacteria but do not kill it.

- **Bactofugation** A process of removing 99 per cent of micro-organism in milk by centrifugal force.

- **Balance** An instrument for weighing.

- **Balanced ration** The ration which provides an animal with the proper amount, proportion and variety of all the required nutrients to keep the animal in its form to perform best in respect of production and health.

- **Balanitis** Inflammation of glans penis.

- **Balanoposthitis** Inflammation of both glans penis and prepuce.

- **Balantidium** A ciliated, protozoan parasite. It can cause scouring in pigs.

- **Balm** A soothing or healing medicine.

- **Balooning degeneration** Isolation of cells of epidermis following intracellularoedema and vacuolation.

- **Band** A strip which constricts or binds a part.

- **Bandages and Bandaging** The application of bandages to veterinary patients is bandaging given protection aginst flies and the infective agent which these carry. Bandages may be needed for support and to reduce tension on the skin. Bandages are made in the form of either single or double roller. Bandage is a long strip of fabric rolled up from one end only.

- **Bang's disease** See Brucellosis.

- **Barbiturates** Derivatives of barbituric acid (Malonyturea). They include wide range of very vlauable sedative, hypnotic or anesthetic agents.

- **Barium** Chemical element.

- **Barium sulphate** being opaque to X-rays is given by the mouth prior to a radiographic examination for diagnositic purposes.

- **Barium sulphide** is sometimes used as a depilatory for the site of surgical operations.

- **Barley hulls** The outer covering of grains i.e. barley.

- **Barn** A farm building used for housing animals and for storage of hay, grain, etc.
- **Barrier** An obstruction.
- **Barrow** A castrated male pig.
- **Bartonella** A genus of bacillus—like microorganisms.
- **Bartonellosis** Infection with *Bartonella* organisms, which occasionally occurs in dogs and cattle.
- **Basis** Fundamental part of an object.
- **Basophil** A granulocyte that readily takes up basic dye.
- **Basophilic stippling** Erythrocyte that shows blue staining, basophilic granules scattered throughout.
- **Battery system** A method of keeping pullets incages.
- **BCG vaccine** A live, attenuated strain of *Mycobacterium bovis* used to provide immunity to tuberculosis.
- **Bed sores** A sore caused by malnutrition of tissues due to prolonged pressure of the body against bedding as seen in long illness.
- **Beef** Meat of adult cattle.
- **Beet molasses** Apart from cane sugar, beet is also utilised for the manufacture of sugar, the product is known as beet sugar.
- **Beet pulp** A fibrous by-product of beet sugar industry.
- **Behavior** All of a person's total activity.
- **Belladonna** is the common name for the deadly night shade flower.
- **Belly** The abdomen.
- **Benign** New growth of cells that not metatise to other organs and also do not infiltrate into the tissue.
- **Benzamine lactate** is another name for eucaine, important group of compounds used as local anaesthetics.
- **Benzene Hexachloride** An insecticide BHC is the common abbreviation.
- **Benzocaine** is a white powder, with soothing properties, used as a sedative for inflamed and painful surfaces.
- **Benzoic acid** is an antiseptic substance used for inflammatory conditions of the urinary system.
- **Benzyl Benzoate** is a useful drug for treating mange in dogs and horses.
- **Benzylpenicillin** This antibiotic is bacteriocide, active

against Gram-positve bacteria, and given by parenteral or intramammary injection.

■ **Beriberi** Disease caused by the deficiency of Thiamine (Vitamin B1)

■ **Berseem** (*Trifolium alexandrinum*) Also called Egyptian clover; a good rabi leguminous fodder with high protein content, rich in phosphate and calcium and easily digestible.

■ **Beta** Second letter of the Greek alphabet. β.

■ **Betamethasone** A corticosteriod.

■ **Bicarbonate of soda** or baking soda, is one of the most useful alkalies both for internal and external application.

■ **Bifurcate** Divided into two branches.

■ **Big head disease** See Bran disease.

■ **Bigneck disease** See Goitre.

■ **Bilateral** Having two sides; pertaining to both sides.

■ **Bile** A greenish-yellow fluid formed in the liver, stored in the gall bladder (except in the horse which has no gall bladder), and secreted via bile duct into the upper small intestine. It functions in digestion.

■ **Bile salts** Bile salts are combinations of bile acids with the amino acids which increase the absorption of fat.

■ **Bilharziasis** (Schistosomiasis) parasitic disease caused by *Scistosoma spp* i.e. a blood fluke infection.

■ **Biliary fever** Syn Canine piroplasmosis.

■ **Biliousness** Severe vomiting, thirst, occasional diarrhoea and refusal to food.

■ **Bilirubin** A bile pigment produced by breakdown of heme and reduction of biliverdin.

■ **Binary fission** The cell elongates or enlarges, a cell wall develops across the middle, and the two cells separate completely.

■ **Binocular** Pertaining to both eyes.

■ **Binomial** Composed of two terms.

■ **Bio** Life, living.

■ **Bioassays** Refer to assay techniques which are used for determining the concentrations of pharmacologically active substances.

■ **Bioavailability** Refers to the proportion of the active drug in a formulation that has been absorbed and therefore available to exert its pharmacological effect.

■ **Bioequivalence** This term is equivalence of bioavailability and hence of biological activity of two products having the same active principle but different formulations.

■ **Biological half-life** The time required for a biological system, such as a human or an animal, to eliminate by natural process half the amount of a substance (such as radioactive material) that has entered it.

■ **Biological value** The efficiency with which a protein furnishes the proper proportions and amounts of the essential amino acids.

■ **Biomass** Total weight of all living organisms in an ecosystem.

■ **Biophysics** Application of the knowledge of physics to the study of living things.

■ **Biopsy** Removal and examination of tissue from the living individual.

■ **Biosynthesis** Process of formation of a chemical substance by a living cell.

■ **Biotechnology** The application of biology, engineering and micro-electronics for increasing human resources.

■ **Biotics** The functions and qualities peculiar to living organism.

■ **Biotin** Water soluble vitamin of B-complex. Widely distributed in natural foods like egg yolk, kidney, liver, and yeast.

■ **Biotoxin** A poisonous substance produced by a living organism.

■ **Birth** See parturition.

■ **Bites** Looked upon as infected wounds.

■ **Biting Louse** an external parasite bites and sucks blood of animals.

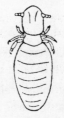

BITING LOUSE

■ **Bitters** The term used for non-toxic amounts of

substances having a bitter taste.

- **Black Disease** (Infectious necrotic hepatitis) is an acute fatal toxaemic disease of sheep, cattle caused by the toxin of *Clostridium novyi*.

- **Black Tongue** Caused by diet deficient in nicotinic acid. Symptoms include discoloration of the tongue, a foul odour from the mouth, ulceration, loss of appetite.

- **Black water fever** is a popular name for Texas fever, which is caused by a piroplasmal parasiate.

- **Blackhead of turkeys** Fatal disease of young turkeys caused by a protozoan parasite—*Histomonas meleegridis*, which is carried into the body by the worms—*Heterakis gallinae*.

- **Blackleg** Blackleg is an acute, infectious disease caused by *Clostridium Chauvoei* and characterized by inflammation of muscles, severe toxaemia and a high mortality. Syn. Black Quarter.

- **Bladder** Thick walled muscular sac serves as reservoir for urine/Bile.

- **Blastocyst** An early embryonic stage, about the seventh day after fertilization.

- **Bleeder** An animal that bleeds easier than normal i.e. one that has hemophilia.

- **Bleeding or Haemorrhage** may be classified according to the vessel or vessels from which it escapes.

- **Blepharitis** Inflammation of eyelids.

- **Blindness** Loss of vision.

- **Blister** A thick vesicle on the skin containing watery fluid or serum caused by burn or other injury.

- **Bloat** Syn Tympanites, Accumulation of gases in the rumen and reticulum.

- **Blocky** Refers to a deep, wide, and low-set animal.

- **Blood** is a red, slightly alkaline fluid which serves as a carrier of nutrients from the digestive system to the various tissues, transports oxygen from the lungs and carbon dioxide to the lungs, carries hormones from the endocrine glands, maintains a correct water balance in the body.

- **Blood brain barrier** Cell membranes that allow some substances to pass form the blood to the brain but restrict others.

■ **Blood meal** Blood which has been dried firstly by passing live steam until the temperature reaches 100°C, the process ensures sterilization and causes blood to clot. It is then drained, pressed to expel occuluded serum, dried again by steam heating and finally ground. The compound contains about 80 per cent protein but deficient in leucine.

■ **Bloodtransfusion** is used in veterinary practice in cases of haemorrhage and shock, and to alesser extent as part of the treatment of certain infectious diseases. Cattle, donor and recipient are usually in the same herd. Blood is collected from the jugular or other vein by means of a suitable needle and syringe, is allowed to flow into a sterilised bottle containing sodium citrate solution.

■ **Blows** Distention of the caecum in the rabbit as a result of excessive gas formation.

■ **Blue bottle flies** Its 'maggots' live on decomposing flesh, and sometimes on skin wounds in sheep.

■ **Blue Comb** See Pullet disease.

■ **Blue nose of horses** It is a photosensetization in horses which occurs due to feeding of spring horse.

■ **Bluetongue** Bluetongue is an infectious disease of sheep and occasionally cattle, caused by a virus and transmitted by insect vectors.

■ **Boar** A sexually mature uncastrated male animal in swine.

■ **Body** the trunk, or animal frame with its organs.

■ **Boil/furuncle** Focal area of suppurative inflammation of skin which involves a hair follicle or sebaceous gland.

■ **Bolus** A roughly spherical mass of food which has been chewed and mixed with saliva ready for swallowing or large tablet form.

■ **Bomb calorimeter** An instrument used for determining the gross energy content of a material.

■ **Bone** It is a mineralised connective tissue and its composition varies greatly with age and site.

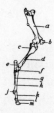

BONES OF HIND LEG

■ **Bone marrow** A highly vascular, cellular substance in the central cavity of some bones. The site of synthesis of erythrocytes, granulocytes and platelets.

■ **Bone pinning** A method of treating fractures wherein a stainless steel pin is introduced into the narrow space to keep the two broken pieces in alignment and to help in healing.

■ **Boophilus** a genus of ticks primarily parasite on cattle.

■ **Boracic or Boric Acid** is found in or is prepared from borax, is a popular but inefficient antiseptic.

■ **Borna disease** Infectious encephalo—myelitis of horses caused by virus.

■ **Borogluconate** The salt of calcium used in solution for intravenous or subcutaneous injection in cases of hypocalcaemia.

■ **Bot flies** Belong to oestrus family of flies, their maggots (larvae) are parasite on horse, sheep etc.

■ **Botrimycosis** A disease caused by staphylococcus which produces fibrous tissue (granulation tissue) with pus in the centre.

■ **Botulism** An infection due to intake of the toxins produce [1] by the bacterium— *Clostridium botulinum.*

■ **Boughs** Solid instruments which are inserted into the natural passages of the body either for purpose of dilatation or for medication.

■ **Bouquet** A structure resembling a cluster of flowers.

■ **Bovine** Pertaining to cattle and buffaloe.

■ **Bovine Farcy** This disease of cattle characterized by purulent lymphangitis and lymphadenitis and is caused by *Nocardia sp.*

■ **Bovine Malignant Catarrh** (BMC)—is an acute, highly fatal, infectious disease of cattle caused by a virus. It is characterized by the development of a catarrhal inflammation of the upper respiratory tract and encephalitis.

■ **Bowel** The lower end of the intestine joined to the ileum. Very little absorption of nutrients occurs in the bowel it is here that water is taken up into the blood.

■ **Brachial** is a word meaning 'belonging to the upper arm'.

■ **Brachy** short.

■ **Bracken poisoning** The eating of bracken by horses, cattle or sheep may lead to serious illness and death.

■ **Brady** Slow.

■ **Bradycardia** Heart action at a reduced rate.

■ **Bradytocia** parturition.

■ **Brain** The brain and the spinal cord together form what is called the *central nervous system*. The principal parts of the brain are— Cerebrum, Brain-stem and Cerebellum.

■ **Bran** The pericarp or seed coat of grain removed during processing.

■ **Bran disease** Osteodystrophia fibrosa, Big head disease, Miller's disease—caused by diet rich in phosphorus and deficient in calcium.

■ **Bran itch** The American name for sarcoptic mange in cattle.

■ **Branch** Offshoot form a main stem.

■ **Branding** A mark of identification embossed on the skin/horn/hoof of the cattle with hot iron die or with chemicals.

■ **Brandy** Alcohol.

■ **Braxy** Braxy is an acute infectious disease of sheep caused by Clostridium septicum and is characterized by inflammation of the abomasal wall, toxaemia and a high mortality rate.

■ **Breasts** Mammary Gland.

■ **Breathing** Respiration.

■ **Breathlessness** Difficulty in breathing.

■ **Breed** A group of animals having common origin and possessing certain distinguishing characters not common to other animals of the same species.

■ **Breed cross** Offspring of a mating between two different breeds.

■ **Breeding** The science and art of bringing improvement in animals through selection and proper mating system.

■ **Breeding chute** A wooden or metal enclosure which

holds a cow or she-buffalo for mating purpose during breeding.

■ **Breeding index** The term is applied to the average number of services per conception in a daily herd.

■ **Breeding value** The genetic ability of an animal to secrete milk, lay eggs.

■ **Bright blindness** Bracken poisoning in sheep or progressive degeneration of retina.

■ **Brightfield microscope** A microscope that uses visible light for illumination.

■ **Brine** A solution containing salt in dissolved condition in water.

■ **Brisket disease** High altitude disease in cattle in which there is oedema of subcutaneous tissue of neck jaws and brisket.

■ **Broilers** Good quality table fowls of either sex about 10–12 weeks old and weighing 2–4 lbs.

■ **Broken wind** syn 'Heaves' A disease in horses characterised by chronic alveloar emphysema.

■ **Bromatology** Refers to science of foods.

■ **Bronchiolitis** Inflammation of very small bronchial tubes.

■ **Bronchitis** Inflammation of bronchie.

■ **Bronchoconstrictor agent** Refers to an agent that is able to produce constriction of the bronchi.

■ **Bronchodilator agent** Refers to an agent that produces dilatation of the bronchi.

■ **Brooder** is an equipment used for providing artificial warmth at controlled temperature for the artificial rearing of chicks.

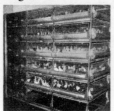

BROODER

■ **Bronchus or bronchial** tube, is the name to tubes into which the windpipe(trachea) divides.

■ **Brow** The forehead.

■ **Brown** A reddish yellow color.

■ **Brucellosis** (Bang's disease) The disease of cattle caused by infection with *Br. abortus* is characterized by abortion late in pregnancy and a subsequent high rate of infertility.

■ **Bruise** Injury by striking or pressing without breaking the skin, causing a subcutaneous haemorrhage.

■ **Bruising** Involve only the deeper layers of the skin or the damage may extend to underlying muscles. Bleeding from injured blood vessels.

■ **Bruit and Murmur** are words used to describe several abnormal sounds heard in connection with the heart, arteries, and veins on asucultation.

■ **BSP clearance test** Bromosulphaline dye clearance test used to determine the functions of liver.

■ **Buccal** Pertaining to the cheeks or mouth cavity.

■ **Buffalo** Belongs to the order Artiodactyle, sub-order ruminantia, family Bovidae, tribe Bovini. Within the Bovini, the distinguishing groups are Bovina (cattle), Bubalina (Asian buffalo).

■ **Buffalo pox** A contagious disease of buffaloes infective agent is distinct from cowpox virus.

■ **Buffer** A substance that tends is stabilize the pH of a solution.

■ **Buffer fat** The fat in milk, butter or any pure milk product.

■ **Buffy coat** The layer of leucocytes, thrombocytes, and nucleated erythrocytes that collects immediately above the erythrocytes in a centrifuged blood.

■ **Bull** A sexually mature uncastrated male bovine.

■ **Bullock** A castrated bull.

■ **Bump** Method of determining pregnancy during the last few months of gestation.

■ **Burdizzo Emasculator** An instrument frequently used in India for castrating bulls.

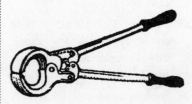

BURDIZZO CASTRATOR

■ **Burna disease** Infections encephalo myelitis of horses caused by virus.

- **Burns and Scalds** Former is cuased by dry heat and the latter by moist heat their lesions and the treatment of these are similar.

- **Burnt colour** Colour which appears after over-heating of milk, usually brownish-black.

- **Burro** A donkey or an ass.

- **Bursa** A sac or sac-like cavity.

- **Bursa** Fluid-filled sac or saclike.

- **Bursa of Fabricius** A lymphoid organ in birds having similar role in immunity to that of the Thymus in mammals.

- **Bursal disease** Infectious bursal disease of poultry.

- **Bursitis** means inflammation within a bursa.

- **Buss disease** Sproadic bovine encephalomyelitis caused by chlamydia sp. and characterized by inflammation of endothelium.

- **Butter** It is obtained from churning sweet or sour cream or obtained by churning curd (dahi).

- **Butter** milk By-product obtaining after the removal of butter from curd by churning or otherwise, also known as lassi or chhach.

- **Butter oil** Fat concentrate obtained from butter or cream after the removal of all the water and SNF.

- **Butter tub**(butter churn) A vessel to agitate the cream, generally a cylinder rotated on a horizontal axis.

- **Butterine** A product composed of 40 per cent milk fat, 40 per cent vegetable fat, 1 per cent milk solids, salt and added Vitamin A and D.

- **Buttock** Either of the two fleshy prominences formed by the gluteal muscles on the lower part of the back.

- **Butyric acid** One of the volatile fatty acids with the formula $CH_2CH_2Ch_2$ COOH.

- **Butyrometer** Specially designed bottle for testing fat in milk or cream.

- **B.Vet. C** British Veterinary Codex

- **By-product** A general term applied to all materials other than the desired product in any manufacturing process.

- **Byre** A cow house.

❑

■ **C.C.B.P.** Contagious Caprine Pleuro Pneumonia disease caused by *Mycoplasma sp* in goats and sheep.

■ **C.R.D.** Chronic Respiratory Disease of chickens caused by *Mycoplasma sp.*

■ **C.V.H.** Canine Virus Hepatitis.

■ **Ca** Chemical symbol, calcium

■ **Cachexia** Extreme weakness and anaemia.

■ **Cadmium** chemical element

■ **Caecum** A blind pouch, open only at one end, in vertebrates, present at the junction of small and large intestine.

■ **Caesarean** section means the removal of the unborn young from the dam by surgical incision into the walls of the abdomen and the uterus, which are afterwards sutured.

■ **Caffeine** Central nervous system stimulant, $C_8H_{10}N_4O_2$, from coffee, tea.

■ **Cake** The residual product left after extraction of oil by mechanical means from mature linseed, groundnut etc.

■ **Calamine, or Carbonate of zinc** is mild astringent used to protect and soothe the irritated skin and used in the form of calamine lotion.

■ **Calciferol** (Vitamin D) Formed by the action of ultraviolet radiation on ergosterol.

■ **Calcification** Deposition of calcium salts in tissues other than bone.

■ **Calcinosis** See Manchester wasting disease.

■ **Calcite** Calcium carbonate, $CaCO_3$, with hexagonal crystallisation, an acceptable source of Ca.

■ **Calcium supplements** These may consist of bone meal, bone flour, ground limestone, or chalk.

■ **Calculi** Are stones or concretions containing salts.

■ **Calculus** A stone which gets formed in tissue like kidney and gall bladder.

■ **Calf** The young ones of any species of cattle, sexually immature, generally upto six months of age.

- **Calf crop** The number, or percentage, of calves produced within a herd in a given year.

- **Calf Diphtheria** A disease of below six months old calves due to *Fusiformis necrophorus*.

- **Calf pneumonia** Virus pneumonia of calves. Mycoplasma and chlamydia are other infective agents which may cause pneumonia.

- **Calf scours** Bacterial diarrhoea caused by Escherichia coli.

- **Calf starter** A special feedingstuff designed for young calves. Dried whey is normally a prominent constituent.

- **Calf-rearing** *In dairy herds*, only bull calves being kept for breeding.

- **Callosity** means thickening of the skin, usually accompanied by loss of hair and a dulling of sensation.

- **Callus** is the lump of new bone that is laid down during the first 2 or 3 weeks after fracture, around the broken ends of the bone.

- **Calomel** mercuric subchloride Calomel is a purgative having a special action on the bile-mechanism of the liver.

- **Calorie** (small) The amount of energy as heat required to raise one gram of water to 1°C (precisely from 14.5° to 15.5°C). This is equivalent to 4.185 g.

- **Calorimeter** An instrument for measuring energy. Parturition or giving birth to calf.

- **Camphor** A ketone derived from the Asian tree Cinnamomum camphora or produced synthetically, used topically as an antipruritic.

- **Canal** Relatively narrow tubular passage or channel.

- **Cancer** A malignant, invasive cellular tumor that has the capability of spreading throughout the body or body parts.

- **Candida albicans** The name of a fungus which gives rise to a disease Candidiasis / Moniliasis in man and animals.

- **Canine** the dog family, including dogs, wolves, jackals, and others.

- **Canine adenovirus infection** Canine virus hepatitis.

- **Canine babesiosis (Piroplasmosis)** also called tick fever. It is due to a blood parasite, *Babesia canis*.

- **Canine distemper** A viral disease of dogs.

- **Canine rickettsiosis** A tick-borne fever caused by *Rickettsia canis*.

- **Canine tooth** Dog tooth of mammals, well developed in carnivores, absent in many herbivores like rabbit, hare, rat, squirrel; present on either side of each jaw in between the incisors and premolars, some times enlarged to tusks as in wild boar.

- **Canine viral hepatitis** is also known as Rubarth's disease or Hepatitis contagiosa canis, Infectious canine hepatitis caused by a virus.

- **Canker** An ulceration, especially of the tip.

- **Canker of the ear** Discharge from the ear.

- **Canker of the foot** A chronic hypertrophic condition of the foot of horse.

- **Cannibalism** This is a vice seen in chicken where the birds pick at each other and cause injury.

- **Cannula** A tube for insertion ito a duct or cavity.

- **Cans** A common trade term for metal containers for milk.

- **Cap** A protective covering for the head or for a similar structure.

- **Capacity** the power to hold, retain, or contain, or the ability to absorb.

- **Caponisation** Castration of poultry.

- **Caprine** Refers to the goat.

- **Caps** capsule

- **Capsid** The protein coat of a virus that surrounds the nucleic acid.

- **Capsule** An outer, viscous covering on some bacteria composed of a polysaccharide or polypeptide.

- **Capsule** is tasteless, readily swallowed, and disintegrates rapidly in the stomach.

- **Caramel** (or burnt sugar) An amorphous brittle brown substance prepared by heating cane sugar under controlled conditions. Used as a colouring and flavouring agent in dairy and food industries.

■ **Carbohydrates** Organic compounds consisting of carbon, hydrogen, and oxygen.

■ **Carbolic acid or Phenol** is a coal-tar antiseptic. When applied to the skin in strong solution it causes death of those cells on the surface and paralyses the superficial sensory nerves.

■ **Carbon** Chemical element symbol.

■ **Carbon dioxide** is formed by the tissues, taken up by the blood, exchanged for oxygen in the lungs, and expired from them with each breath.

■ **Carbon monoxide** poisoning may result from gas and solid fule heating systems in the home when there is an inadequate supply of air.

■ **Carbon tetrachloride** is used against liver flukes and round worms in animals.

■ **Carbuncle** Focal area of suppurative inflammation of skin in which there is discharge of pus into the exterior through several sinus tracts.

■ **Carcass** The body of dead animal.

■ **Carcinogenic** Cancer producing.

■ **Carcinoma** is a type of malignant growth.

■ **Cardia** is the upper opening of the stomach at which the oesophagus terminates.

■ **Cardiac cycle** One contraction relaxing cycle of heart.

■ **Cardiac Drugs** Drugs employed in the treatment of heart disease.

■ **Cardiography** is the process by which graphic records can be made of the heart's action.

■ **Cardiology** is the name given to a study of the heart and heart diseases.

■ **Cardiovascular** Pertaining to the heart and blood vessels.

■ **Caries** Decay of teeth in which enamel is decalcified followed by softening and discolouration.

■ **Carminative** Refers to a substance which is having the property of assisting the expulsion of gas from the stomach and intestines.

■ **Carnivorous** Meat-eating animals including dogs, cats etc.

■ **Carotene** A yellow organic compound that is a precursor of vitamin A.

■ **Carpals** These are six short bones arranged in two rows between the radius and ulna above and metacarpal bones below.

■ **Carrangeena** A product from carrageen (Irish moss) seaweed, used as stabilizer in ice cream.

■ **Carrier** An individual who harbours a pathogen but exhibits no signs of illness.

■ **Cartilage** These are nonvascular pliable strong structures and form supporting framework of articulating surfaces of bones and certain organs of the body.

■ **Caruncle** A small fleshy protuberance, which may be a normal anatomical part.

■ **Case** Particular instance of a disease.

■ **Caseation** Conversion of tissue to a necrosed cheesy mass. Often seen in tuberculosis.

■ **Casein** Casein is a group name for the dominant class of proteins in milk.

■ **Caseous lymphadentitis** Chronic disease of the sheep and goat, characterised by the formation of nodules containing a cheesy pus occurring in the lymphatic glands, lungs, skin, or other organs.

■ **Cast** A positive copy of an object.

■ **Castration** Removal or severence of spermatic chord of testes

■ **Casualty** An accident, an accidental wound death.

■ **Catabolism** The conversion of complex substances into more simple compounds by living cells. Destructive metabolism.

■ **Catalo** (Cattalo) A crossbed animal produced by mating American Bison with domestic cattle.

■ **Catalyst** A substance that speeds up the rate of a chemical reaction but is not itself used up in the reaction.

■ **Cataract** Opacity of the Crystalline lens of the eye.

■ **Catarrh** Inflammation of mucous membranes, particularly those of the air passages.

■ **Catch** Term used by livestock men to indicate that conception has taken place after breeding.

■ **Catechu** A powerful astringent extracted form leaves and twigs of ourouparia gambir.

■ **Catgut** A sterile strand obtained from collagen derived form healthy mammal, used as a surgical ligature.

■ **Cathartic** Refers to a drug that is able to produce emptying of the bowels.

■ **Cathetars** Tubes used for passing along the urethra in order to draw off urine.

■ **Catheter** A tubular, flexible instrument passed, through body channels for with drawl of fluids form.

■ **Cathode** The negative electrode from which electrons are emitted.

■ **Cattle** Refers to the mature bovine animal.

■ **Cattle crush** Syn. Crush.

■ **Cattle plague** which is also known as Rinderpest, is an acute, specific, inoculable, and febrile disease of cattle.

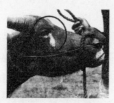

CATTLE PLAGUE

■ **Caudal** Towards tail end

■ **Caustics** are used to burn diseased or healthy tissues acting by chemical energy.

■ **Cavity** A hollow place or space, or a potential space, within the body.

■ **Cecum** It is a blind sac which has a length of about 75cm and is a part of large intestine.

■ **Cell** The building blocks of the body containing a cell wall surrounding a bit of protoplasm and contains a nucleus and cytoplasm.

■ **Cell culture** Animal or plant cells grown in vitro.

■ **Cell wall** The outer covering of most bacterial, fungal, algal, and plant cells.

■ **Cellulose** The main carbohydrate substance making up the cell membrane of plants. It is digested and made available to ruminants by the action of microorganisms in the rumen.

■ **Cement** A substance that produces a solid union between two surfaces.

■ **Center** The middle point of a body.

■ **Centi** Hundred.

■ **Centigrade** Having 100 gradations as the Celsius scale; abbreviated C.

■ **Central** Nervous System (CNS) This comprises the brain and spinal cord.

■ **Cephal** Head

■ **Cephalexin** Oral cephalosporin used in the treatment of pneumococcal.

■ **Cephalomycins** Refers to a series of antibiotics which have been similar to the cephalosporins but deri-ved from *Streptomyces* species.

■ **Cephalosporins** Refer to a series of antibiotics, the first to which were isolated from *Cephalosporium acremonium*.

■ **Ceramics** The modeling and processing of objects made of clay or similar materials.

■ **Cercaria** A free-swimming larva of trematodes.

■ **Cereals** Such as wheat, barley, oats, rye, maize, millets, and rice are all rich in startch and comparatively poor in proteins and minerals poor in calcium but richer in phosphorus.

■ **Cerebellum** A subdivision of brain which lies behind the forebrain and above the brainstem. It controls the muscle movements for smoothly integrated body movements.

■ **Cerebral** Anoxia When the supply of oxygen to the brain is reduced for any reason.

■ **Cerebral hemispheres** A pair of structures in vertebrate forebrain that contain the centres concerned with major senses, voluntary muscle activities, and higher brain function, such as language and memory.

■ **Cerebrospinal fluid** Fluid which fills the cavity inside vertebrate brain and spinal cord.

■ **Ceroid** Oxidised product of unsaturated fatty acids accumulated in the tissues.

■ **Cervical** Pertaining to neck region. Cervical vertebrae are the vertebrae of neck.

■ **Cervix** The firm muscular opening of the uterus which opens out to the vagina.

■ **Cestoda** (Tapeworm) A class of phylum Platyhelminthes including mostly endo-parasitic forms with no digestive tract but with hooks and suckers for attachment and other parasitic adaptations and a complex life-cycle, e.g. *Taenia*.

■ **Cetavlon** Syn Cetrimide.

■ **Cetrimide** An antiseptic of value in wound treatment and for cleaning cows' udders and teats.

■ **CF** Crude fibre.

■ **Chain** A collection of objects linked to gether in a linear fashion.

■ **Chamber** An enclosed space.

■ **Character** A term used to designate any form, function, or feature of an individual.

■ **Charcoal** (Bone black) is the product obtained by charring (partial burning) of bones in closed retorts (a container generally of glass with a long tube, in which substances are decomposed by heat).

■ **Chastek paralysis** Paralysis in Foxes, Minks and Cats due to thiamine (Vit B_1) deficiency.

■ **Cheeks** They form the lateral walls of the mouth.

■ **Cheese** Cheese is the fresh or ripened product obtained after coagulation and whey separation of milk, cream, partly skimmed milk, butter milk or a mixture of these proteins.

■ **Cheese vat** The container used for the production of cheese curd.

■ **Cheilitis** Inflammation of lips

■ **Chelating agents** are substances which have the property of binding divalent metal ions to form stable, soluble complexes.

■ **Chelation** Chelation is a process in which an organic grouping combines with or "binds" another substance, usually a metallic ion.

■ **Chemical** A substance composed of chemical elements, or obtained by chemical processes.

■ **Chemist** An expert in chemistry or pharmacist.

■ **Chemistry** The science of the interactions of atoms and molecules.

■ **Chemosurgery** Destruction of tissue by chemical means for therapeutic purpose.

- **Chemotherapy** Treatment of disease by chemical agents.
- **Chest, or Thorax** is a conical cavity, with the apex directed forwards. The base is formed by the diaphragm while the sides are formed by the ribs, sternum, and vertebrae.
- **Chicks** New born fowl or bird.
- **Chlamydia** Small round or ovoid bacteria.
- **Chloral hydrate** Usually called Chloral, substance produced by prolonged action between alcohol and chlorine, dissolves rapidly in water, acts as a hypnotic, or a depressant to the central nervous system.
- **Chloramines** These are combinations of chlorine and ammonia and are fairly stable powered disinfectants.
- **Chloramphenicol** A broad spectrum bacteriostatic antibiotic.
- **Chlorodyne** is very similar in composition to the compound tincture of chloroform and morphia.
- **Chloroform** is a colourless, mobile, inflammable liquid. When given by the mouth, acts as a carminative, antispasmodic, and anodyne, inhaled by the nostrils it induces general anaesthesia in all animals.
- **Chlorophyll** The green colouring matter present in growing plants.
- **Chloroquine** An anti malarial.
- **Chlorpromazine** Hydrochloride used for preanaesthetic medication, also as a tranquilliser.
- **Chocolate milk** A drink having whole or skimmed milk, cocoa and sugar with permissible flavour and preservative.
- **Choking** means an obstruction to respiration, obstruction to the passage of food through the pharynx and oesophagus, either partial or complete.
- **Cholagogue** Refers to a substance that promotes the flow of bile form the gall bladder into the duodenum.
- **Cholangitis** Inflammation of bile duct.
- **Cholecystitis** Inflammation of gall bladder. Choleliths Biliary concretions i.e. gall stones.

■ **Choleretics** Refer to the substance that stimulate the secretion of bile e.g. bile salts themselves taken by mouth, or cholice acid by intravenous injection.

■ **Cholesterol** A mono-unsaturated, secondary alcohol sterol.

■ **Choline** One of the B vitamins.

■ **Cholinergic** or parasympathomimetic drug is one which augments or duplicates the effects of stimulating a parasympathetic nerve.

■ **Cholinergic nerves** A cholinergic nerve ending is one which iberates acetylcholine.

■ **Chondr(o)** Cartilage.

■ **Chondral** Pertaining to cartilage.

■ **Chondrectomy** Surgical removal of a cartilage.

■ **Chondrification** Deposition of calcium salts in a preformed matrix prepared by chondrocytes.

■ **Chopped** Reduced in particle size by cutting.

■ **Chordata** A phylum of the animal kingdom comprising all animals having a noto-chord during some developmental stage.

■ **Chorea** A disease of central nervous system caused by bacterial or organic degeneration. Most common in dogs following canine distemper characterized by irregular, jerkey involuntary muscular movements.

■ **Chord** Cord.

■ **Chorditis** Inflammation of vocal or spermatic cord.

■ **Chorioamnionitis** Bacterial infection of foetal membrane.

■ **Chorioptic Mange** (Tail Mange of cattle)

■ **Choroid** is the middle of the three coats of the eye, and consists of the blood vessels.

■ **Chromatolysis** Dissolution of Nissle substance of neuron.

■ **Chromocyte** Any colored cell or pigmented corpuscle.

■ **Chromosomal** aberration Any irregularities in chromosome number or morphology of a species.

■ **Chromosome** Cell orgnelles carrying the hereditary material DNA, occur in pairs in somatic cells.

- **Chronic** Slow prolonged reaction.
- **Chuni** Chuni means 'Churna'. The compound consists primarily of the broken pieces of endosperm including germ and a portion of husks obtained as by-product during the processing of pulse grains for human consumption.
- **Churning** The violent agitation and beating of cream in the butter making process.
- **Chyle** is the name given to the partly digested food as it passes down the small intestine.
- **Chylocele** Accumulation of lymphatic fluid in the tunica vaginalis.
- **Chyme** is the partly digested food passed from the stomach into the first part of the small intestine.
- **Cicatrix** A scar.
- **Cinchona** the dried bark of the stem or root of various trees of the genus cinchona; it is the source of quinine.
- **Cine** Movement.
- **Cinematography** the taking of motion pictures.
- **CIP** Clean-in-place. A method of cleaning dairy equipment and sanitary pipelines by pumping and circulating washing solutions without dismantling them.
- **Circum** Around.
- **Circumscribed** Bounded or limited; confined to a limited space.
- **Cirrhosis** Chronic inflammation of liver.
- **Cistern** Closed space serving as a reservoir for fluid.
- **Citrate** A slat of citric acid.
- **Clarified Ghee** Butter from which water has been removed by heat, the salt and curd being allowed to settle and the fat filtered off. Known as *ghee* in India.
- **Clarified milk** Milk from which visible foreign matter is removed to improve its quality.
- **Clavicle** This bone is found embedded in brachiocephalic muscle in front of shoulder joint.
- **Claws** Most insects have two horny claws derived from the last segment of the tarsus.
- **Clean environment** A controlled atmosphere under which standard pasteurized product is packaged into

standard containers resulting in longer refrigerated storage.

■ **Cleavage** Division into distinct parts, early successive splitting of a fertilized ovum into smaller cells.

■ **Cleft** A fissure in a bone

■ **Click** a brief, sharp sound.

■ **Climate** Prevailing weather conditions in a particular area.

■ **Climax** The period of greatest intensity, as in the course of a disease.

■ **Clinical** Word is used to denote anything associated with the practical study of a sick person, or animal.

■ **Clitoris** (glands clitoridis) The small organ lying just inside and at the bottom of the vulvar opening which is the female counterpart of the male penis.

■ **Cloaca** Posterior part of the alimentary canal into which the urinary and reproductive ducts open, in birds, reptiles, amphibians and many fishes.

■ **Clock** A device for measuring time.

■ **Clomiphene citrate** A fertility drug that stimulates ovulation through the release of gonadotrophins from the pituitary gland.

■ **Clone** A population of cells that are identical to the parent cell.

■ **Clonic spasms** Intermittent spasms

■ **Closebreeding** The mating of close relatives such as parents and offspring or full brothers and full sisters.

■ **Closed herd** (or flock) A herd or flock where no outside breeding animals are used.

■ **Clostridium** A genus of anaerobe spore-bearing bacteria of ovoid, spindle, or club shape.

■ **Clotted milk** Milk in which thick agglomerates of protein and fat are formed.

■ **Clotting of blood** This is a very complex process. Jelly-like clot consistss of minute threads of filaments or fibrin, which are enmeshed red blood corpuscles, white blood-cells, and platelets. When the injury giving rise to the bleeding occurs, *thromboplastin* is released from the damaged tissue and from the platelets, and reacts with circulating *prothrombin* and calcium to form *thrombin*. This reacts to produce the fibrin.

■ **Cloudburst** This term is used when spontaneous discharge of a cloudy uterine fluid occurs around the expected time of parturition in animal that are suffering from pseudopregnancy.

■ **Cloudy swelling** Disturbance of protein metabolism in which cell swells and cytoplasm becomes more granular.

■ **Cloxacillin** A semisynthetic penicillin, sodium salt is used in treating staphylococci infections.

■ **Coagulating enzymes** Milk clotting enzymes.

■ **Coagulation** Another name for clotting.

■ **Coat** The half covering of the body of an animal.

■ **Cobalamine** (Vitamin B_{12}) Cobalt containing vitamin required by many organisms.

■ **Cobalt** is one of the mineral elements known to be essential to normal health, but required in minute amounts.

■ **Cocci** The spherical bacteria are called cocci.

■ **Coccidiomycosis** is a fungal disease, involving chiefly the lymph nodes, and giving rise to tumour lesions.

■ **Coccidiosis** A protozoal disease of animals and birds caused by the genus Eimeria and Isospora etc.

■ **Coccidiostat** Medicines which are used for the prevention of coccidia.

■ **Coccobacillus** A bacterium that is an oval rod.

■ **Coccygeal vertebrae** These are incomplete vertebrae and form the skeleton of the tail.

■ **Cochlea** Part of membranous labyrinth (inner ear) concerned in the reception of sound with analysis of its pitch.

■ **Cocks** Male fowls used for breeding.

■ **Cod** Liver Oil is one fo the most valuable sources of vitamins A and D available for animal feeding.

■ **Code** A set of rules for regulating conduct.

■ **Codeine** is one of the active principles of opium, and is used as the phosphate of codeine to check severe coughing in bronchitis.

■ **Coefficient** An expression of the change or effect produced by variation in certain factors, or of the ratio between two different quantities.

■ **Coefficient** of digestibility The percentage value of a food nutrient that has been absorbed.

■ **Coenzyme** A partner required by some enzymes to produce enzymatic activity.

■ **Cofactors** Additional component besides the enzyme and substrate required before the reaction are called cofactors.

■ **Coitus** Copulation of male and female, a term generally used in connection with mammals.

■ **Colibacillosis** Commonest disease of newborn caused by *E.coli*. Manifested by diarrhoea, septicaemia (bacteraemia) and sudden death.

■ **Colic** A vague term to designate any form of abdominal pain especially in horses.

■ **Coliform test** A test for estimating coliform bacteria in a milk sample.

■ **Coliforms** Aerobic or facultatively anaerobic, and a Gram-negative, nonspore-formating, rod-shaped bacteria that ferment lactose with acid and gas formation .

■ **Colitis** Inflammatilon of the colon.

■ **Collagen** The main supportive protein of connective tissue.

■ **Collapse** To fall unconscious due to disease, attack or injury.

■ **Colon** Large intestine of vertebrates, excluding the narrower terminal rectum.

■ **Colony** A clone of bacterial cells on a solid medium that is visible to the naked eye.

■ **Colostrum** The first milk after giving birth to young in mammals. It contains large amounts of antibodies and vitamins.

■ **Colour blindness** (Red green) Genetically controlled defect in which one cannot distinguish between red and green colour.

■ **Colt** A young male horse.

■ **Coma** Unconsciousness.

■ **Comb** In healthy poultry, this should be bright red and well developed. It is on the head of the bird.

■ **Combustion** The combination of substances with oxygen accompanied by the liberation of heat.

■ **Commensalism** A system of interaction in which two organisms live in association and one is benefited while the other is neither benefited nor harmed.

■ **Commensals** Micro-organisms found on the skin or within the body which normally do not produce disease.

■ **Commissure** means a joining, and is a term applied to strands of nerve fibres that join one side of the brain to the other.

■ **Communicable disease** Any disease that can be spread from one host to another.

■ **Complaint** A disease, symptom or disorder.

■ **Complementary genes** Genes which interact (work together) to produce a trait they don't produce when not together.

■ **Complete ration** A single feed mixture into which has been included all of the dietary essentials, except water of given class of livestock.

■ **Complex** The sum or combination of various things, like or unlike, as a complex of symptoms.

■ **Complexion** The color and appearance of the skin of the face.

■ **Compliance** Expression of the measure of ability to do so.

■ **Complication** A disease (s) concurrent with another disease.

■ **Compost** Decomposing organic matter.

■ **Compound** A substance composed of two or more different chemical elements.

■ **Compound feeds** A number of different ingredients (including major minerals, trace elements, vitamins and other additives) mixed and blended in appropriate proportions to provide properly balanced diets for all types of stock at every stage of growth and development. In some cases, e.g. ruminants, compound feeds are technically designed when fed without further mixing with cereals, to supplement natural foods (e.g. grass or rough ages) available on the farm. In such cases the compound feed is frequently given a name defining its purpose, e.g. for balancing straw, grass, kale, silage, etc.

■ **Compound light microscope** An instrument with two sets of lenses that uses visible light as the source of illumination.

■ **Compression** Act of pressing upon or together; the state of being pressed together.

■ **Compressor** Any agent by which compression may be achieved.

■ **Concave** Rounded and somewhat depressed or hollowed out.

■ **Concentrate** Feeds having crude fibre less than 18 per cent while T.D.N. is over 60 per cent on air dry basis.

■ **Concept** The image of a thing held in the mind.

■ **Conception** Getting pregnant.

■ **Concretions** Compact or solidified unorganised masses of material which may or may not originate within the body.

■ **Condensed milk** A product obtained by evaporating water from whole or skimmed milk partly or fully,

with or without the addition of sugar.

■ **Condenser** A lens system located below the microscope stage that directs light rays through the specimen.

■ **Condom** A sheath or cover to be worn over the penis in coitus to prevent impregnation or infection.

■ **Condyle** A cylindirical articular eminence at distal extremity of bone.

■ **Confection** Preparation of sweets from milk or its by-products.

■ **Confinement** Restraint within a specific area.

■ **Conformation** The shape and arrangement of the different body parts of an animal.

■ **Congenital** A trait acquired before birth and present at birth.

■ **Congestion** Increased amount of blood in venous side of vascular system.

■ **Conjunctiva** This is a thin transparent membrane which covers the front portion of sclera and cornea .

■ **Conjunctivitis** Inflammation of conjunctiva.

■ **Connective tissues** These include white fibrous tissue, yellow elastic tissue, reticular tissue, adipose tissue, cartilage and bone.

■ **Conscious** Capable of responding to sensory stimuli.

■ **Constant** Not falling; remaining unaltered.

■ **Constipation** When the motility of intestine is reduced the faeces are dry, hard and of small bulk and are passed at infrequent intervals.

■ **Consultation** Deliberation by two or more physicians about diagnosis or treatment in a particular case.

■ **Consumption** The act of consuming, or the process of being consumed.

■ **Contact** Mutual touching of two bodies or persons.

■ **Contagious** Ability to spread by contact.

■ **Contagious** abortion of cattle Syn Brucellosis.

■ **Contagious caprine pleuropneumonia** A disease of goats, caused by Mycoplasma.

■ **Contaminant** Something that causes contamination.

■ **Contamination** The soiling or making inferior by contact.

■ **Contra** Opposed.

■ **Contraceptives** Products used for preventing bitches, etc. coming on heat.

■ **Control, controlled experiment** In any scientifically conducted experiment or field trial, the results of treatment of one group of animals are compared with results in another, untreated, group. Animals in the untreated group are known as 'the controls'.

■ **Convex** Having a rounded, somewhat elevated surface.

■ **Convulsions** Widespread spasms involving whole body.

■ **Cooked flavour** Flavour defect in milk due to overheating.

■ **Cooperia** A genus of parasitic nematodes sometimes found in the small intestine of ruminants.

■ **Coordination** The harmonious functioning of interrelated organs and parts.

■ **Copper** is used in veterinary medicine only as the sulphate, which is also known as 'bluestone' and 'blue vitriol'. Internally, it is astringent, irritant and emetic. Sometimes used as an antidote to phosphorus poisoning. Externally, it is an astringent and caustic. Copper is also one fo the trace elements which is essential in the nutrition of animals.

■ **Copra meal** The product is what remains after the dried edible portion of coconuts have been subjected to fat extraction and round. The relatively low quality of its protein and its relative high content of fibre restrict use in rations for swine and poultry.

■ **Coprophagia** The eating of faeces by the animals. Cornea Transparent part of the eye of vertebrates, overlying iris and lens.

■ **Corns** A horny projection of the epidermis usually with a central core formed specially on the toes or feet.

■ **Coronary** is a term applied to several structures in the body encircling an organ in the manner of a crown.

■ **Coronavirus** This genus of viruses includes the infectious bronchitis group and transmissible gastro-enteritis of pigs.

■ **Corpus luteum** A yellow glandular mass in the ovary formed by an ovarian follicle that has matured and discharged its ovum. The corpus luteum secretes progesterone.

■ **Correlation** A measure of how two traits tend to move together.

■ **Cortical granule** Specialized secretory vesicles lying just below the plasma membrane of the egg, that fuse and release their contents immediately after fertilization.

■ **Corticosteroids** These are the steroid hormones which are synthesized and secreted by the adrenal cortex.

■ **Corticotrophin** The hormone from the anterior lobe of the pituitary gland which controls the secretion by the adrenal gland of corticoid hormones.

■ **Cortisol** A steriod from the adrenal gland.

■ **Cortisone** A hormone from the cortex of the adrenal gland. Cortisone raises the sugar content of the blood and the glycogen content of the liver, among other actions.

- **Coryza** Respiratory disease in poultry.

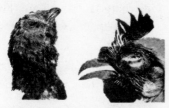

CONTAGIOUS CORYZA

- **Cotton seed hulls** The outer protective covering of cotton seeds.

- **Cotton seed oil cake** Residue which remains after mechanical pressing of clean cotton seed composed, principally of the kernel with such unavoidable portions of the hull and fibre as may be left in course of expression of oil.

- **Cotyledon** The cotyledon is a rosette of minute folds at the point of attachment of the placenta to the dam's tissues

- **Cough** Coughing is a reflex act initiated by irritation of the respiratory mucosa of the air passages.

- **Count** Numerical computation or indication.

- **Counterirritants** ounterirritants are drugs that are employed to irritate the intact skin in order to relieve pain originating from the underlying tissues.

- **Courtship** Special behaviour of animals in seeking mates.

- **Coverglass** Thin glass plate that covers a mounted microscopical object or a culture.

- **Coverslip** Coverglass.

- **Cow** A mature female cattle, more commonly referred to *Bos taurus* or *Bos indicus*.

- **Cowper's gland** A gland of male reproductive ducts of mammals whose acidic secretion is a part of the seminal fluid.

- **Cowpox** It is a contagious skin disease of cattle characterized by the appearance of typical pox lesions on the teats and udder caused by virus.

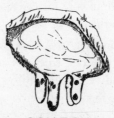

COWPOX

- **Coxalgia** means pain in the hip-joint.

- **CP** Crude protein.

- **Cramp** Painful involuntary contraction of a muscle.

- **Crani** Skull.
- **Cranial** Towards the head end
- **Crazy chick disease** Nervous disease in chicks due to the deficiency of Vitamin E (Syn Avaian encepholomalacia).
- **Cream** A portion of milk rich in fat.
- **Creatinine** A nitrogenous compound arising from protein metabolism and excreted in the urine.
- **Creatinuria** Presence of excessive creatinine in urine due to excessive endogenous breakdown of muscle in the urine.
- **Crenation** Shrinkage of cells in a hypertonic solution with formation of irregular margin and number of prickly points.
- **Crepitations** is the name applied to certain sounds which occur along with the normal sounds of breathing, as heard by auscultation, in various diseases of the lungs.
- **Crop** Dilatation of the oesophagus at the base of the neck in poultry.
- **Croup** Region of the sacrum.
- **Crucial** Severe and decisive.

- **Cruciform** Cross-shaped.
- **Crude fibre** The more fibrous, less digestible portion of a feed. Consists primarily of cellulose, hemicellulose and lignin.
- **Crumbles** Pellets reduced to a granular texture.
- **Crush** An appliance constructed of wood or tubular steel, and used for holding cattle.
- **Cryosurgery** Destruction of unwanted tissue of a tumour by the use of very low temperatures. For example, a metal rod, cooled in liquid nitrogen to—196°C, may be applied to the tumour.
- **Crypt(o)** Concealed.
- **Cryptococcosis** An yeast—*Cryptococcus* neoformans causing a disease in animals.
- **Cryptorchidism** When one or both testes fail to descend from the abdominal cavity into the scrotum.
- **Crystal** A naturally produced angular solid of definite form.
- **Crystalluria** Presence of crystals in the urine.
- **Cud** Ruminating a bolus of previously eaten food which has been regurgitated by a

ruminant animal for further chewing.

■ **Culling** Rejecting unproductive or undesirable birds or animals.

■ **Culture** Media on which microorganisms grow i.e growth outside the body in a medium.

■ **Curd** The solid part of milk that separates from the liquid in the making of cheese.

■ **Curled toe paralysis** Paralysis caused in birds due to Riboflavin (Vitamin B_2) deficiency.

■ **Currete or curet** A spoon-shaped instrument for cleaning a diseased surface.

■ **Cutaneous** Pertains to skin.

■ **Cuticle** Nonliving outer covering of helminths.

■ **Cyandies** are salts of hydrocyanic or prussic acid. They are all highly poisonous.

■ **Cyanocobalamine** Same as vitamin B_{12}.

■ **Cyanosis** Cyanosis is a bluish dis-colouration of the skin, conjunctivae and visible mucosae.

■ **Cycle** Succession or recurring series or events.

■ **Cyst** A sac with a distinct wall containing fluid or other material.

■ **Cystic ovaries** Presence of cysts in the ovaries e.g. follicular cyst or leutinising cyst or atretic follicles.

■ **Cystine** One of the nonessential amino acids.

■ **Cystitis** Inflammation of the urinary bladder.

■ **Cyt(o)** A cell.

■ **Cytogenetics** The study of chromosomes.

■ **Cytokines** Small proteins released from human cells in response to bacterial infection.

■ **Cytology** The study of the origin, structure and function of cells.

■ **Cytoplasm** The protoplasm of the cell outside the nucleus but within the cell membrane.

■ **Cytotoxin** Bacterial toxins that kill or alter the functions of host cells.

❏

- **D.V.M.** Doctor of Veterinary Medicine.

- **Dahi** *See* curd.

- **Dairy** A farm where milk is produced, more commonly, a place where milk and milk products are processed and offered for sale.

- **Dairying** The business of operating a dairy, including distribution and selling of milk and its products.

- **Dandruff** Syn. Pityriasis. It is a condition characterized by the presence of Bran like scales on the skin surface.

- **D.C.I.** Drug Controller of India

- **DDT** The common abbreviation for dichlorodiphenyl trichlo-rethane, a potent paracitiside, lethal to fleas, lice, flies, etc.

- **Deafness** Unable to listen.

- **Death** The termination of vital processes in the organism.

- **Debeaking** Clippng off a small portion of the tip of the beak.

- **Debility** Weakness.

- **Debris** Devitalized tissue or foreign matter.

- **Decidua** Is mucous membrane (endometrium) lining the uterus in the thickened and modified form it acquires during pregnancy in many mammals.

- **Decolorizing agent** A solution used in the process of removing a stain.

- **Decongestants** Agents which remove congestion.

- **Decortication** Removal of the bark, hull, husk or shell from a plant seed, or root.

- **Dectyl** A digit or finger.

- **Deep litter for cattle** This is system. Straw, shavings, and sawdust can be used. Warmth given off as a result of the fermentation taking place in the litter makes for cow.

- **Deep litter system of raising poultry** Chopped straw wood shavings or saw dust are used for spreading on the floor 4" thick and the birds live on such a pen.

- **Defaecation** Passing out of dung.
- **Defective** Imperfect.
- **Deferium** A state of violent excitement or emotion.
- **Deficiency** A lack or shortage ; a condition characterized by presence of less than normal.
- **Deficiency disease** A disease in which there is decreased to its deficient level in diet or due to metabolic disturbances.
- **Definitive host** Refers to the "Host' (or animal) in which the adult parasite lives.
- **Defluorinated** Having had the fluorine content reduced to a level which is nontoxic under normal use.

Deformity Distortion of any part or general disfigurement of the body.

- **Deglutition** Swallowing
- **Degnele Disease** Disease of bovines which brings about necrosis of the extremities (hoofs, ear, tail etc.).
- **Degree** Grade or rank.
- **Dehorning** Removal of horns from cattle surgically or chemically.

- **Dehulling** Dehulling is the process of removing the outer coat of grain, nuts and some fruits.
- **Dehydration** Loss of water from the body.
- **Delicious** pleasant, toothsome, palatable.
- **Delivery** Syn parturition.
- **Demodectic** Mange or Follicular Mange Mites of Demodex spp. infest hair follicles of all species of domestic animals but most commonly dogs.
- **Demulcents** Demulcent drugs are a group of water-soluble compounds which tend to coat over irritated or abraded tissue surfaces to protect the underlying cells from irritating contacts.
- **Demyelinating diseases** Diseases affecting the nervous system whereby there is destruction of the myelin sheath—a covering of the nerve fibre.
- **Dengue** Syn Three-day sickness.
- **Dentine** Main constituent of teeth.
- **Dentition** Form and arrangement of teeth in the vertebrates.

■ **Denture** Complement of teeth, either natural or artificial.

■ **Deodorant** Deodorant is anything, usually a chemical, which removes or masks odors.

■ **Deposit** Sediment or dregs.

■ **Depraved appetite** Syn appetite.

■ **Depression** A hollow or depressed area.

■ **Dermatitis** Inflammation of the skin.

■ **Dermatology** The study, diagnosis and treatment of the skin and its diseases.

■ **Dermatophytosis** Superficial infection of skin by dermatophytes (Trichophyton, Microsporon and epidermophyton genera).

■ **Dermis** The inner portion of the skin.

■ **Desi** Indigenous.

■ **Desiccate** To dry completely.

■ **Desiccation** The removal of water.

■ **Designed** Premediated, intentional.

■ **Detergents** are substances which cleanse, and many are among the best wetting agents.

■ **Detoxication** Means destruction of a toxic compound, or more usually, alteration of a chemical group to produce a non-toxic prdouct.

■ **Dettol** A proprietary nontoxic antiseptic of much value for skin lesions and obstetrical work. (Antiseptics)

■ **Device** Something contrived for a specific purpose.

■ **Dextrin** An intermediate polysaccharide product ob-tained during starch hy-drolosis.

■ **Dextrose** is another name for purified, grape sugar or glucose.

■ **Diabetes insipidus, or Polyuria** is a condition in which there is secretion an excessively large quantity of urine of low specific gravity.

■ **Diabetes mellitus** is a condition in which an excess of sugar (glucose) is found in the urine.

■ **Diagnose** to identify or recognize a disease.

■ **Diagnosis** Judgement of a particular or specific abnormal state of health.

- **Diagram** A graphic representation.

- **Dialysis** A techniqe for separating compounds with small molecules from compounds with large molecules by selective diffusion through a semipermeable membrane.

- **Diaphragm** A sheet of tissue, part muscle, part tendon, covered by serous membrane, separating cavities of thorax from cavity of abdomen. Present only in mammals.

- **Diaphragmatic** Hernia Herniation of a portion of the reticulum through a diaphragmatic rupture.

- **Diarrhoea** An intestinal disorder characterized by abnormal frequency and fluidity of fecal evacuations.

- **Diastole** means the relaxation of a hollow organ. The term is applied in particular to the heart, to indicate the resting period that occurs between the beats while the blood is flowing into the organ.

- **Diathermy** is a process by which electric currents can be passed into the deeper parts of the body so as to produce internal warmth and relieve pain.

- **Dichlorophen** A drug of value against tapeworms in the dog.

- **Dicoumarol** A chemical compound found in spoiled sweet clover and lespedeza hays.

- **Die** a form used in the construction of something.

- **Dieldrin** An insecticide of particular value against the maggot-fly of sheep.

- **Diet** A regulated selection of a feed ingredient or mixture of ingredients including water, which is consumed by animals on a prescribed schedule.

- **Dietetics** the science of diet and nutrition.

- **Digestion** The processes involved in the conversion of feed into absorbable forms.

- **Digestion** coefficient (Coefficient of digestibility) The difference between the nutrients consumed and the nutrients excreted expressed as a percentage.

- **Digestive system** See Alimentary canal.

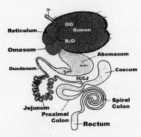

DIGESTIVE SYSTEM

- **Digitoxin** An alkaloid obtained from *Digitalis*, used in the treatment of certain heart conditions.

- **Dihybrid** An individual that is heterozygous for two pairs of genes such as individual AaBb.

- **Dilator** A structure (muscle) that dilates, or an instrument used to dilate.

- **Diodone** A contrast medium used in radiography of the kidneys.

- **Diphtheria** An acute contagious disease caused by the diphtheria bacillus (*Corynebacterium diphtheria*) which gain entry through respiratory passsage.

- **Diplegia** means extensive paralysis on both sides of the body.

- **Diploid** Normal paired (2n) chromosoes in body cells.

- **Diplopia** Double vision; seeing one object as two.

- **Dips and dipping** Dips are tanks containing a solution of insecticides or acaricides, to remove ectoparasites and prevent further infestation by them.

- **Disaccharide** Any one of the several so-called compound sugars which yield two monosaccharide molecules upon hydrolysis.

- **Discharge** An excretion or substance evacuated.

- **Disease** Any deviation from healthy state

- **Disinfectant** Disinfectant or germicide is a substance used to destroy bacteria or other infective organisms.

- **Dislocation** The displacement of any part from the normal position especially with reference to joints.

- **Disorder** Abnormality of function.

- **Dispermic** An ovum fertilized by two spermatozoa rather than the usual one.

- **Disperse** To scatter the component parts.

- **Displaced** Dislodge, oust.

- **Displacement** Removal to an abnormal location or position.

- **Dissolve** To cause a substance to pass into solution.
- **Distal** remote; farther from any point of reference.
- **Distemper** is a name applied to a specific virus disease with high fever.
- **Distress** Physical or mental anguish or suffering.
- **Diuretics** Refers to the substances that increase the secretion of urine.
- **Diverticulum** Circumscribed pouch or sac occurring normally.
- **Dizygote twin** More than one ovum is fertilized and develop into offspring.
- **DM** Dry matter.
- **DNA** Di-oxyribonucleic acid
- **Docking** Removal of tail.
- **Doctor** Practitioner of the he-aling arts, as one graduated from a college of medicine, osteopathy, dentistry, veterinary medicine, and licensed to practice.
- **Dominant** Describes a gene that covers up the expression of its allele when paired together in body cells.
- **Donor** An organism that supplies living tissue to be used in another body. As a person who furnishes blood for transfusion, or an organ.
- **Donor cell** A cell that gives DNA to a recipient cell in recombination.
- **Dorsal** /superior Directed upwards towards the back.
- **Dose** the quantity to be administered at one time, as a specified amount of medication.
- **Douche** Irrigation.
- **Doughy** When the structure pits on pressure as in oedema.
- **Dourine** A venereal disease of horses caused by *Trypanosoma equiperdum.*

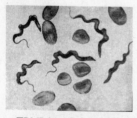

TRYPANOSOMA

- **Downer** cow syndrome Milk fever cases which do not respond to calcium therapy.
- **D.P.C.O.** Drug Price Control Order.
- **DPT vaccine** A combined vaccine used to provide active

immunity, containing diphtheria, tetanus toxoids and killed Bordetella pertussis cells.

■ **Drainage** Systematic withdrawal of fluids and discharges from a wound sore, or cavity.

■ **Drenching** The giving of liquid medicines to animals through bottle or bamboo pipe.

■ **Dressing** Any of various materials used for covering and protecting a wound.

■ **Drip** The slow, drop-by-drop infusion of a liquid.

■ **Drop** Minute sphere of liquid as it hangs or falls.

■ **Dropper** A pipe or tube for dispensing liquid in drops.

■ **Dropsy** Accumulation of serous fluid in the abdominal cavity. Also known as Ascites.

■ **Drowning** Suffocation and death resulting form filling of the lungs with water or other substance or fluid.

■ **Drug** The word drug has been defined by the Pure Food and **Drug** Act to the medicine and preparations recognized in the United States Pharmacopieia for internal and external use, for the cure, mitigation, or prevention of disease of either man or other animals.

■ **Drug antagonism** It refers to the opposing action of two drugs on the same tissue.

■ **Drug** Idiosyncrasy Drug idiosyncrasy or drug allergy is an unusual type of tissue response to the presence of a drug.

■ **Drug synergism** Synergism refers to the enhancement of a tissue response by the concomitant use of two or more drugs.

■ **Dry cow** A cow which has stopped giving milk.

■ **Dry period** A period between the end of one lactation and the beginning of another.

■ **Drying off** The act of making a cow dry before she is due to calve again.

■ **Dual-purpose breed** Cattle bred and kept for two purposes—for milk and draught (work) or milk and producing meat.

■ **Duct** Passage with well defined walls.

■ **Ductless glands** Endocrine glands.

■ **Dumb** Unable to speak; mute.

■ **Dummy syndrome** Condition in which the animal remains standing and is able to move but does not respond at all to external stimuli is usually referred to as the 'dummy' syndrome.

■ **Dung** The faeces or excreta of an animal.

■ **Duodenum** Upper portion of small intestine starting with the end of stomach and ending with jejunum.

■ **Duplication** The process in which a chromosome is attached to a portion of its own homologous chromosome, thus giving duplicate genes.

■ **Duramater** This is the outermost strong and tough fibrous covering of brain and spinal cord.

■ **Dusting powders** Inert substances used for protective action, are readily and harmlessly disposed off by the tissues of the body.

■ **Dyad** Two sister chromatids that are joined together (synapsed) giving a tetrad.

■ **Dysentery** A disease characterized by frequent, watery stools containing blood and mucus.

■ **Dysfunction** Disturbance, impairment, or abnormality of functioning of an organ.

■ **Dyspepsia** Impairment of the normal digestive function.

■ **Dysphagia** Condition in which animal feels difficulty in eating.

■ **Dysponea** Difficulty in breathing.

■ **Dystokia** Difficulty in parturition (giving birth)

■ **Dystrophy** Defective or faulty nutrition or development.

■ **Dysuria** means the absence of urine.

❑

E/e

■ **E. Coli** This is an abbreviation for Escherichia coli, formerly known as Bacillus coli—a normal inhabitant of the alimentary canal in most mammals. E. Coli scours are common in new-born lambs and often fatal.

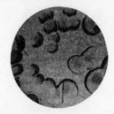

ESCHERICHIA COLI

■ **E.D.$_{50}$** Median effective dose; a dose that produces its effects in 50% of a population.

■ **E.S.R.** Erythrocyte sedimentation rate.

■ **Ear** This is an organ associated with hearing and equilibrium.

■ **Ear** canker of A popular term applied somewhat indiscriminately to any inflammation of the lining of external ear.

■ **East coast fever** Theileria parva, which spends part of its life-history in cattle and part in ticks. Animal becomes dull, listless, loses appetite, and runs a high fever. Lymph nodes become enlarged.

■ **Echinococosis** Invasion of the tissue with the larvae of the tapeworm called *Echinococus granulosus.*

■ **Echo** Resonant repetition of a sound heard on auscultation of the chest.

■ **Eclampsia** Lactation tetany of mares caused by hypocalcaemia which is characterized by convulsions.

■ **Ecobolic** Drugs which cause contraction of uterine muscle.

■ **Ecology** The study of the interrelationships between organisms and their natural environment, both living and nonliving.

■ **Ecthyma** A localized inflammation of skin characterised by the formation of pustules.

■ **Ecto** is a perfix meaning on the outside.

■ **Ectoderm** The outermost of the three primitive germ layers of the embryo.

■ **Eczema** Inflammatory condition of skin in which there is formation of vesicles or scales / crust (dry or moist).

■ **Edema** is another spelling of oedema.

■ **EEE** Eastern equine encephalomyelitis.

■ **Effect** The result produced by an action.

■ **Efferent** Conveying away from a center, as an efferent nerve.

■ **Efficiency** Ratio (FER) This is an index of efficiency expressed in terms of kg. of feed consumed per dozen of eggs produced in layers or per kg. of weight gain in meat in broilers.

■ **Egg bound** A condition in laying poultry in which an egg or eggs may be formed in the oviduct normally but the hen is unable to discharge it.

■ **Eimeria** A genus of sporozoa (order Coccidia).

■ **Eisenmenger complex** Hypoplasia of the aorta.

■ **Ejaculation** A process to release semen by the male at mating.

■ **Elastic** capable of resuming normal shape after distortion.

■ **Elbow** Joint Postero-lateral aspect of the shaft of radius and anterior surface of the body of ulna.

■ **Electro-cardiogram (ECG)** is a record of the variations in electric potential wh;ich occur in the heart as it contracts and relaxes.

■ **Electrocautery** An apparatus for cauterizing tissue by means of a platinum wire heated by electric current.

■ **Electrocution** Exposure to high-voltage electric currents causing sudden nervous shock with temporary unconsciousness or immediate death.

■ **Electroencephalogram (EEG)** A tracing or graph of the electrical activity of the brain.

■ **Electrolyte** A substance that dissociates into ions fused in solution.

■ **Electron** A negatively charged particle in motion around the nucleus of an atom.

■ **Electron microscope** These costly and complex instruments have made it possible to study and photograph viruses, bacteriophages, and the structure of bacteria.

■ **Electro-therapy** High frequency currents About 5 to 20 minutes daily or for shorter periods twice daily. Faradic currents are used to produce rhythmic muscular contractions in the treatment of muscles.

■ **Electuary** A soft paste made by compounding drugs with treacle, sugar or honey and rubbed on the tongue.

■ **Element** Any one of the fundamental atoms of which all matter is composed.

■ **Eleo** Oil.

■ **Elimination** The act of expulsion especially expulsion from the body.

■ **Elisa** (enzyme-linked immunosorbent assay) Assay for detection or quantitation of an antibody or antigen using a ligand (e.g. an anti-immunoglobulin) conjugated to an enzyme which changes the color of a substrate.

■ **Elixir** The term used for an alcoholic solution of a medicament.

■ **Emaciated** An excessively thin condition of the body.

■ **Embedding** Fixation of tissue in a firm medium.

■ **Embolism** means the plugging of a small blood-vessel by a piece of some material that has been carried into it from larger vessels.

■ **Embryo** A term for the developing young during about the first one quarter of the gestation period or pregnancy.

■ **Embryo transfer** Transfer of a fertilized egg at 4–8 cell stage (embryo) obtained from a donor female (generally genetically superior) to a recipient female.

■ **Embryogenesis** Formation of organs during foetal life.

■ **Embryology** Study of prenatal development of an individual.

■ **Emesis** means vomiting.

■ **Emetics** An emetic is a drug that produces vomition.

■ **Emollients** Emollients are usually fatty substances applied to soften the skin.

■ **Emphysema** Abnormal distension of the lung caused by rupture of alveolar walls with or without escape of air into the interstitial tissue.

■ **Emphysematous** The structure is puffy and swollen, and moves and crackles under pressure.

■ **Empyema** Accumulation of pus in a preformed body cavity (Peritoneal or pleural cavity).

■ **Emulsify** To disperse small drops of one liquid into another liquid.

■ **Enamel** the white, compact, and very hard substance covering and protecting the dentin of a tooth crown.

■ **Encephalitis** Inflammation of brain.

■ **Encephalomalacia** Softening of brain tissue.

■ **Encysted** The term is applied to parasites, collection of pus, fluid etc which are shut off from the surrounding structures by a ring of dense fibrous tissue or by a membrane.

■ **End artery** Terminal branches of any artery are called end arteries.

■ **End(o)** Within; inward.

■ **Endemic disease** A disease that is constantly present in a certain population.

■ **Ending** termination.

■ **Endo** is a prefix meaning situated inside.

■ **Endocarditis** Inflammation of the endocardium of heart.

■ **Endochondral osteogenesis** Formation of bone in the cartilaginous tissue.

■ **Endocrine** glands These are ductless glands or glands of internal secretion.

■ **Endogenous** Originating from within the organism.

■ **Endometrial hyperplasia** Thickening of the endometrial lining due to an overgrowth of mucosal cells.

■ **Endometriosis** A condition in which tissue more or less perfectly resembling the uterine mucous membrane (the endometrium) and containing typical endometrial granular and stromal elements occurs aberrantly in various locations in the pelvic cavity.

■ **Endometritis** Inflammation of the endometrium.

■ **Endometrium** The mucous membrane that lines the uterus.

■ **Endoparasites** Internal parasites such as worms and coccidia.

■ **Endoscopes** An instrument for examining the interior of a hollow viscous.

■ **Endoskeleton** The cartilaginous and bony skeleton of the body.

■ **Endospore** A resting structure formed inside some bacteria.

■ **Endosteum** The marrow cavity and marrow spaces in a bone are lined by a layer of areolar tissue known as endosteum.

■ **Endothelium** is the membrane lining various vessels and cavities of the body, such as the pleura, pericardium, peritoneum.

■ **Endotoxins** are those toxins which are retained within the bodies of bacateria until the latter die and disinegrate.

■ **Enema** A liquid medicament for injection into the rectum.

■ **Energy** The capacity to perform work.

■ **Ensiling** A process of making silage from fodder.

■ **Entad** Toward a center.

■ **Ental** Inner; central.

■ **Enter(o)** intestines.

■ **Enteritis** Inflammation of the intestines.

■ **Entero** Toxaemia Sheep-Bacterial disease caused by toxins of *Clostridum welchi.*

■ **Enteroliths** Concretions of intestines

■ **Enterostomy** means an operation by which an artificial opening is formed in intestine.

■ **Enteroviruses** A group of smaller viruses pathogenic to animals and causing disease in cattle, pigs and ducks.

■ **Entomology** That branch of biology concerned with the study of insects.

■ **Environment** The sum total of all external influences to which an individual is exposed.

■ **Enzootic** Term applied to the outbreak of a disease among animals in a particular area or district periodically.

■ **Enzootic Ataxia** /Swayback of Lambs Enzootic ataxia is caused by copper deficiency.

■ **Enzootic ovine** abortion is caused by *Chlamydia psittaci.*

■ **Enzootic pneumonia of pigs** Virus Pneumonia of Pigs but the cause is now generally regarded as being *Mycloplasma hyopneumoniae.*

■ **Enzootic pneumonia of sheep** Pasteurellosis, pneumonia of sheep.

■ **Enzymes** Enzymes are organic catalysts, produced only in living cells, which exhibit a high degree of specificity in the substances they activate.

■ **Eosinophilia** An increase in the number of eosinophils in the blood.

■ **Ephedrine** An adrenegic, $C_{10}H_{15}N0$ used as a bronchodilator in the form of the hydrochloride.

■ **Ephemeral fever** Ephemeral fever is an infectious disease of cattle characterized by inflammation of mesodermal tissues as evidenced by muscular shivering, stiffness, lameness and enlargement of the peripheral lymph nodes. The disease is caused by a virus which is transmitted by insect vectors. Or this is known as three day sickness.

■ **Epi**—is a prefix meaning situated on or outside of.

■ **Epidemic** When many people in a given region are attacked by same disease at the same time.

■ **Epidemiology** Relationships of various factors determining the frequency and distribution of diseases.

■ **Epidermis** The outer portion of the skin.

■ **Epididymis** It is a curved elongated structure situated along the caudal border of testis.

■ **Epidural injection** For the introduction of local anesthetic into the epidural space.

■ **Epidural** situated upon or outside the dura mater.

■ **Epilepsy** An attack of alternating tonic and clonic spasms accompanied by loss of consciousness.

■ **Episiotomy** incision of the vulva for obstetric purposes.

■ **Epistasis** Interaction of two or more pairs of genes that are not alleles to produce a phenotype that they don't produce when they occur separately.

■ **Epistaxis** Haemorrhage from the nasal cavity.

■ **Epithelium** is the layer or layers of cells of which skin and mucous membranes are formed.

■ **Epizootic** Widely dispersed, rapidly spreading disease.

■ **Epsom salts** is the popular name for sulphate of magnesium, which is one of the most frequently used saline purgatives.

■ **Equator** An imaginary line encircling a globe or globular.

■ **Equilibrium** A state of balance between opposing forces or influences.

■ **Equine** Refers to the horse.

■ **Equine influenza** This is an infectious respiratory disease caused by a virus and characterized by mild fever and a severe, persistent cough.

■ **Equine Viral Rhinopneumonitis** (EVR) A mild disease of the upper respiratory tract of horses caused by a specific virus which also commonly causes abortion.

■ **Erection** The condition of being rigid and elevated, as erectile tissue when filled with blood.

■ **Ergosterol** One of the sterols which upon exposure to ultraviolet light is converted to vitamin D_2.

■ **Ergot** A toxin produced in sclerotia by the fungus *Claviceps purpurea* that causes ergotism.

■ **Ergot therapy** Drug which stimulates the smooth muscle of uterus.

■ **Ergotism** Poisoning due to ingestion of ergots of Calviceps purpurea.

■ **Erosion** Defect in skin in which there is loss of superficial layer only.

■ **Erotic** Pertaining to sexual love or to lust.

■ **Eructation** Occurs in dorsal sac, passes forward to cardia of the oesophagus in conjunction with reticular relaxation.

■ **Eruption** The act of breaking out, appearing, or becoming visible.

■ **Erysipelas** The major disesease of animals caused by this bacterium with arthritis, laminitis.

■ **Erysipelothrix** A genus of gram-positive bacteria.

■ **Erythema** The redness produced during inflammation.

■ **Erythr(o)** Red.

■ **Erythrocytosis** The increased in erythrocyte count in the blood.

■ **Erythropoiesis** The production of erythrocytes.

■ **Erythromycin** An antibiotic which has a bacteriostatic action against Gram positive organisms.

■ **Esophagus** It is a muscular tube extends from pharynx to stomach.

■ **Essence** Mixture of alcohol with a volatile oil.

■ **Essential amino acids** Amino acids that are needed by animal and cannot be synthesised by them in the amount needed.

■ **Essential dysmenorrhoea** Painful menses due to a functional disturbance and not due to organic factors.

■ **Essential fatty acid** A fatty acid that cannot be synthesised in the body or that cannot be made in sufficient quantities for the body's needs.

■ **Essential** Indispensable; as essential fatty acids.

■ **Ester** A compound formed from an alcohol and an acid by elimination of water, e.g., ethyl acetate.

■ **Estradiol and Estrone** are hormones secreted by the ovary which bring about oestrus and, in late pregnancy, stimulate development of the mammary gland.

■ **Estrogen** The "female" hormone produced by the developing follicle which causes the period of estrus as well as preparing the reproductive tract for pregnancy and bringing about development of the mammary system.

■ **Estrous** The sexual cycle of the female mammal.

■ **Ethambutol** Tuberculostatic agent.

■ **Ether** Colorless, transparent, mobile, very volatile, highly inflammable liquid, $C_2H_5.O.C_2H_5$.

■ **Ether extract** A constituent of a feed that will dissolve in ether. Represents fat and fat-like ingredients.

■ **Ethnic** Pertaining to a social group who share cultural bonds or physical (racial) characteristics.

■ **Ethology** the scientific study of animal behavior, particularly in the natural state.

■ **Ethyl chloride** is a clear colourless liquid, produced by the action of hydrochloric acid upon alcohol, used to produce insensibility for short surface operations, such as the removal of warts or small tumours.

■ **Ethylene** is a colourless inflammable gas which is sometimes used as an anaesthetic in small animals.

■ **Ethylmorphine** Its hydrochloride salt is used as an antitussive and narcotic.

■ **Etiology** Study of the cause of disease.

■ **EU** is a prefix meaning satisfactory or beneficial.

■ **Eunuch** A male deprived of the testes or external genitals.

■ **Euphoria** Bodily comfort, Absence of pain or distress.

■ **Euploid** The occurrence of chromosome numbers in the individual which is a whole-number multiple of the basic or haploid number.

■ **Euthanesia** Euthanesia is the production of quiet, painless death in an animal for humane reasons.

■ **Evacuation** An emptying, the bowels.

■ **Evaporation** The changing of liquid into gas.

■ **Evolution** a developmental process in which an organ or organism becomes more and more complex by differentiation of its parts.

■ **Examination** Inspection or investigation, especially as a means of diagnosing disease.

■ **Exanthema** Skin rash or eruption.

■ **Exanthematous diseases** Diseases which are characterized by skin eruptions are known as exanthematous diseases.

■ **Excipient** means any more or less inert substance added to a prescription in order to make the remedy more suitable form for administration.

■ **Excise** To remove by cutting.

■ **Excitation** An act of irritation or stimulation.

■ **Exciting causes** Actual cause of the disease

- **Exclusion** Shutting out or Elimination.

- **Excoriation** Destruction of small pieces of skin or of mucous membrane, often by chaffing i.e. rubbing.

- **Excreta** The products of excretion—primarily faeces and urine.

- **Exercise** Performance of physical exertion for improvement of health correction of physical deformity.

- **Exhalation** The giving off of watery or other vapor.

- **Exhaustion** Privation of energy with consequent inability to respond to stimuli.

- **Exogenous** Originating from outside of the organism.

- **Exostosis** Bony prominances due to formation of granulation tissue of bone.

- **Exotoxin** A toxin or poisonous substance excreted by bacteria into the culture medium or food i.e. toxins practical outside the body.

- **Expectorant** Drugs which remove secretion /discharge from the respiratory tract.

- **Expectorant** Promoting expectoration.

- **Expectoration** the coughing up and spitting out of material from the lungs, bronchi, and trachea, sputum.

- **Expiration** The act of breathing out, or expelling air form the lungs.

- **Expire** to breathe out, to die.

- **Exposure** The act of laying open, as surgical exposure.

- **External auditory meatus** It is a canal which leads medially towards the middle ear.

- **External ear** Auricle or pinna and external auditory meatus.

- **External** Situated or occurring on the outside.

- **Extra** outside, beyond the scope of, in addition.

- **Extraction** The process or act of pulling or drawing out.

- **Extractor** An instrument for removing a calculus or foreign body.

- **Extracts** Extracts are solids obtained by evaporating the solvent from tinctures or fluid-extracts.

- **Extremity** The distal or terminal portion of elongated or pointed structures.

- **Extrinsic factor** A factor coming from or originating from outside an organism.

- **Exudate** Fluid with a high content of protein and cellular debris which has escaped from blood vessels and has been deposited in tissues.

- **Exudative diathesis** Caused by vitamin-E deficiency in poultry and is characterised by an accumulation of fluid in subcutaneous fatty tissue.

- **Eye** Eyes are the chief organs of vision.

- **Eye ball** It is spherical in shape composed of three coats—fibrous, vascular and nervous.

- **Eye lashes** At the margin of the lids there are stiff hairs, termed cilia or eye lashes.

- **Eye lids** These are two fibrous sheets, attached to the periphery of the orbital margin cover the anterior portion of the eye ball when it is closed.

- **Eyeworms** In cattle *Thelazia* worms are called.

❑

F/f

■ **F.D.A.** Food and drug administration.

■ **F.R.C.S.** Fellow of the Royal College of Surgeons.

■ **F.S.H.** (Follicle stimulating hormone) produced in the anterior pituitary which stimulates the ovarian follicle to develop.

■ **F1 generation** The first filial generation, or the first-generation progeny following the parental, or P1, generation.

■ **F2 generation** The second filial generation, or the second-generation progeny following the parental, or P1, generation.

■ **Facial** Pertaining to the face.

■ **Factor** an agent or element that contributes to the production of result.

■ **Facultative anaerobes** Organisms which can grow in either the presence or absence of oxygen.

■ **Faeces** The excrement of an animal; dung.

■ **Fagopyrism** Photosenstisation caused by fagopyrin present in seeds and mature plant of buckwheat (*Polygonum fagopyrum*).

■ **Falliculogemin** It is the production of fertizable ova.

■ **Falling** Disease of Cattle Characteristic behaviour in falling disease is for cows in apparently normal health to throw up their head, bellow and fall. Death is instantaneous in most cases but some fall and struggle feebly on their sides for a few minutes' and attempts to rise. The condition caused by copper deficiency and taking due to heart failure.

■ **Fallopian tube** The long tortuous tube into which the egg passes after ovulation on its way to the uterus.

■ **False oestrus** Display of oestrus or heat symptoms by a female when she is pregnant or out of season in seasonally polyoestrous animals.

■ **Family** The term used to denote relationship but more often to represent a group of animals having a genetic relationship.

■ **Fang** the root of a tooth.

■ **Farcy** Cutaneous glanders in horses.

■ **Farrowing** The act of parturition in sows—female pigs.

■ **Fascia** A sheet of fibrous tissue occurring beneath the skin and also enveloping glands, vessels, nerves, and forming tendon sheaths.

■ **Fascioliasis** Infestation with liver flukes *Fasciola hepatica.*

■ **Fat** Fats are esters of glycerol and fatty acids such as palmitic and stearic.

■ **Fatal** Causing death.

■ **Fat-Free milk** Milk with most of the fat removed.

■ **Fatigue** When we do some work or activity, its output decreases gradually and a stage comes when the activity cannot be continued any further without having some rest. When the organism feels the necessity of rest, we say that fatigue has set in.

■ **Fattening** This is the deposition of unused energy in the form of fat within the body tissues.

■ **Fatty acid** Any one of several organic compounds containing carbon, hydrogen, and oxygen which combine with glycerol to form fat.

■ **Fatty degeneration** A condition in which there is an excess of fat in the parenchymatous cells of organs such as the liver, heart and kidneys.

■ **Fatty liver** Syndrome in chicken The condition in which excessive amount of fat are present in the liver, kidneys and myocardium.

■ **Fauna** Frequently used to refer to the overall protozoal population present.

■ **Favus** Syn honeycomb ringworm.

■ **Fe** Chemical symbol, iron.

■ **Fear** a normal emotional response, in contrast to anxiety and phobia.

■ **Febrile** Pertaining to fever.

■ **Fecundity** A measure of fertility, such as sperm count or egg count or the number of live offsprings produced by an organism.

■ **Feed** Harvested forages, grass or other processed feeds made from cereals and cereal by-products, used for feeding livestock.

■ **Feed** Feed or feed mixture fortified with extra vitamins and nutrients.

■ **Feedback** The return of some of the output of a system as input so as to exert some control in the process.

■ **Feline enteritis** A specific viral enteritis in cats.

■ **Female genital organs** The organs of female genital system are ovaries, oviducts, uterus, vagina and vulva. Mammary gland considered as an organ accessory to the female reproductive system.

■ **Feminine** Womanly, lady-like.

■ **Femur** It is a cylindrical and largest long bone in the skeleton. It is directed downward and forward. This bone articulates with the hip-bone above to form hip joint and with tibia, fibula and patella below to form the stifle joint.

■ **Feral** Domesticated animals that have reverted to the wild state.

■ **Fermentation** Decomposition of carbohydrates by micro-organisms in the absence of air, i.e., respiration and oxidation do not occur.

■ **Ferrous** Containing iron.

■ **Fertility** The ability to reproduce.

■ **Fertilization** The union of the male and female reproductive cells to initiate the development of a new individual.

■ **Fetal** Pertaining to a fetus.

■ **Fetlock joint** Joint formed by distal end of metacarpal bone and proximal ends of 1st pair of phalanges and proximal sesamoid bones.

■ **Fetus** The developing individual in intra-uterine life after the body parts are formed.

■ **Fever 666** Caused by *Coxiella brunetii* in cattle and man causing batchy nodular lesions in visceral organs.

■ **Fever or pyrexia** A syndrome in which there is rise in body temperature, disturbance in metabolism along with various functional disturbances.

■ **Fibre** This is coarse woody cell walls of mature plants.

■ **Fibrin** is a substance upon which depends the formation of blood clots.

■ **Fibroblast** A flat, irregularly shaped connective tissue cell.

■ **Fibroid** Having a fibrous structure.

■ **Fibroma** is a tumour consisting of fibrous tissue.

■ **Fibropurulent** containing both fibers and pus.

■ **Fibrosis** Formation of fibrous tissue.

■ **Fibrous** High in cellulose and/or lignin content.

■ **Fibrous** Containing fibers.

■ **Fibrous tissue** is one of the most abundant tissues of the body, being found in quantity below the skin, around muscles and less extent between them.

■ **Fibula** This is bone of hind limb and is highly rudimentary in ox.

■ **Field** An area or open space.

■ **Filamenous bacteria** These forms are elongated and threadlike, and some of them are branched.

■ **Filament** a delicate fiber or thread.

■ **Filariasis** is a group of diseases caused by the presence in the body of certain small thread-like Nematode worms, called filariae, which are often found in the bloodstream.

■ **Filled milk** Milk in which butter fat has been replaced wholly, or partly, by vegetable fat or non-dairy fat.

■ **Film** A thin layer or coating.

■ **Filter** a device for eliminating certain elements as particles of certain size from a solution.

■ **First aid** Emergency care and treatment of an injured before complete medical and surgical treatment can be secured.

■ **First meiotic division** The first of two divisions occurring in reductional cell division and resulting in the production of two cells, each of which is haploid, the chromosomes occurring as paired chromatids joined at the centromere.

■ **Fish oil** Oil extracted from undecomposed dried fish.

■ **Fish scrap** Consists mostly of unedible portion like bones and some viscera of fish.

■ **Fission** Reproduction by division of the body into two parts, each of which becomes a complete organism.

- **Fissures** These are the cracks which penetrate more deeply usually in subcutaneous tissue.

- **Fistulous withers** A sinus developing in connection with the withers of the horse.

- **Fits** is another name for convulsive seizures accompanied usually by at least a few seconds of unconsciousness.

- **Flagella** Thin appendages that arise from one or more locations on the surface of a cell and are used for cellular locomotion.

- **Flaked** Rolled or cut into flat pieces.

- **Flap** Mass of a tissue for grafting usually including skin.

- **Flask** A laboratory vessel, usually of glass and with a constricted neck.

- **Flatulance** Distended abdomen due to presence of gas in stomach.

- **Flatus** Gas or air in the gastrointestinal tract.

- **Flavour** A blend of taste and smell sensations evoked by a substance in the mouth.

- **Flavoured milk** Milk standardized to a certain fat percentage to which some flavour such as chocolate and fruit syrup is added.

- **Fleas** They are two winged insects.

- **Fleece** Rot of Sheep Fleece rot of sheep is a dermatitis caused by prolonged wetting of the skin and resulting in matting of the wool by exudate.

- **Flesh** The soft, muscular tissue of the animal body.

- **Flexion** A displacement of the uterus in which the organ is bent so far forward or backward that an acute angle forms between the fundus and the cervix.

- **Flocculation** Loosely aggregated mass of material suspended in or precipitated from a liquid.

- **Flock** A group of birds or sheep.

- **Flora** The plant life present.

- **Flu** Popular name for influenza.

- **Fluctuation** A variation.

- **Fluid** a liquid ; any liquid of the body.

- **Fluid extracts** These are alcoholic or hydroalcoholic extracts of plants.

- **Fluke** A flatworm belonging to the class Trematoda.

■ **Fluorescence** The ability to give off light of one color when exposed to light of another color.

■ **Fluorescence** microscope A microscope that uses an ultraviolet light source to illuminate specimens that will fluoresce.

■ **Fluoroquinolone** Synthetic antibacterial agents that inhibit DNA synthesis.

■ **Flurosis** Chronic disease caused by continuous ingestion of small but toxic amounts of fluorine.

■ **Foaling** Parturition in mares.

■ **Foals** Young horses of either sex until they are one year old. Males are called colt foals and females filly foals.

■ **Foaming** A foam is an "emulsion" of a gas (air) in a liquid.

■ **Fodder** The stalks and leaves of dry crop plants or those of fresh plants given as feed to livestock.

■ **Foetus** A term for the developing young during about the last three quarters of the gestation period or pregnancy.

■ **Fog fever** An allergic reaction to proteins in cattle causing pulmonary emphysema and oedema.

■ **Foil** Metal in the form of extremely thin sheet.

■ **Fold** A thin recurved margin or doubling.

■ **Folic acid(folacin)** A vitamin of the vitamin B complex.

■ **Folium** Leaflike structure.

■ **Follicle** The collection of cells and fluid which take part in the production of the ovum. This is termed the Graaffian follicle just prior to ovulation or rupture of the follicle.

■ **Follicle** cell A layer of cells within an ovarian follicle which surrounds the oocyte(proto-ovum) and provides certain nutrients to it.

■ **Follicle** stimulating hormone (FSH) This is secreted by the anterior lobe of the pituitary gland, and stimulates the development of the Graafian follicles in the ovary and controls the secretion of oestrogens from the ovary.

■ **Folliculitis** Inflammation of follicle.

■ **Folliculoma** Granulous cell tumour.

■ **Follicular mange** is another name for demodectic mange

due to the parasite *Demodex canis*.

■ **Follicular phase** The follicular phase is the pre-ovulatory phase of a woman's reproductive cycle during which the follicle grows and high oestrogen levels cause the uterine lining to grow.

■ **Fomentation** Poultices.

■ **Fomite** A nonliving object that can spread infection.

■ **Foot-and-mouth disease** Foot and mouth disease is an extremely contagious, acute disease of all cloven-footed animals, caused by a virus and characterized by fever and a vesicular eruption in the mouth and on the feet.

■ **Footrot of cattle** Infectious disease of cattle characterized by inflammation of the sensitive tissues of the feet and severe lameness.

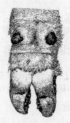

FOOTROT

■ **Forage** Green stuff obtained from the crops raised for the livestock feeding.

■ **Foramen** Natural opening passage especially one into or through a bone.

■ **Forceps** A two-bladed instrument with a handle for compressing or grasping tissues in surgical operations.

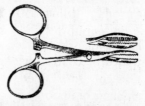

ARTERY FORCEPS

■ **Force** Energy or power.

■ **Forehead** The parts of the face above the eyes.

■ **Formate** A salt of formic acid.

■ **Formula** An expression, direction for preparation or of the composition of.

■ **Fore-milk** The first milk drawn out of the teats at the beginning of milking.

■ **Fortify** Nutritionally, to add one or more nutrients to a feed.

■ **Formalin** is a gaseous body prepared by the oxidation of methyl alcohol. For commercial purposes it is prepared as a solution of 40 per cent strength in water. Formalin is a powerful antiseptic, and has the quality of hardening or fixing the tissues.

■ **Fossa** a trench channel; in anatomy, a hollow.

■ **Foundation** The structure or basis on which something is built.

■ **Fovea** Shallow depression.

■ **Foveola** A minute depression.

■ **Fowl cholera Syn.** Avian pasteurellosis. Haemorrhagic septicaemia of the fowl. This is a contagious disease of fowls.

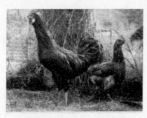

FOWL

■ **Fowl pest** This term usually refers to newcastel disease.

■ **Fowl pox** (Avian contagious epithelioma and Avian Diphtheria) is a virus disease in which wart-like nodules appear on the comb, wattles, eyelids, and openings of the nostrils.

■ **Fowl typhoid** This is an acute infectious disease of fowls caused by the Salmonella gallinarium.

■ **Frambesioma** A rapid structure for giving support to or for immobilizing a part.

■ **Free martin** A masculanised female calf born cotwin with a male and is always sterile.

■ **Freeze drying** Freeze drying is the only reliable method of preserving labile materials and consists of drying the frozen material under high vacuum.

■ **Frequency** The number of occurrences.

■ **Freshen** Act of starting the lactating cycle directly after calving.

■ **Fructose** A six-carbon sugar $C_6H_{12}O_6$—differing from glucose in containing a keto group (on C_2) instead of an aldehyde group.

■ **Fruit** Matured ovary of a plant, including the seed and its envelops.

■ **Full feed** A term usually given to fattening cattle when given all of the concentrated feed they will consume without going off feed.

■ **Full sibs** Full-brothers and full-sisters.

■ **Fumarate** A salt of fumaric acid.

■ **Fumigation** Is a means of disinfection by the use of the vapour of powerful antiseptics, insecticides etc.

■ **Function** Special normal, or proper action of any part or organ.

■ **Functional dysmenorrhoea** Painful menses due to functional disturbances and not due to organic factors such as growths, inflammation or anatomy.

■ **Fungi** Fungi are a group of micro-organisms comprising of molds and yeasts.

■ **Fungicide** Substance which kills fungi is called fungicide.

■ **Funiculitis** The Infla-mmation of spermatic cord.

■ **Furazolidone** A drug used in the treatment of Blackhead and Hexamitiasis.

■ **Fusiform** Spindle-shaped.

❑

- **G Gravity** the unit of force exerted upon a body during acceleration and deceleration.

- **Gait** Movements of the limbs can be expressed in terms of rate, range, force and direction of movement.

- **Galactose** A sugar which is an isomer of glucose. Commonly known as fruit sugar.

- **Gall bladder** A membranous 'sac lying next to the liver of all animals (except the horse) in which bile is stored.

- **Gall-Stones** which are also known as *Biliary calculi*, concretions which are formed in the gall-bladder or in the bileducts of the liver.

- **Gama globulin** Is a protein fraction of blood serum which contains the antibodies against certain bacteria and viruses.

- **Gamete** A reproductive cell (sex cell, germ cell) of either sex; e.g. sperm or an egg (ovum).

- **Gametogenesis** The process by which gametes are formed in the gonads of male or female.

- **Gammexane** products contain the gamma isomer of benzene hexachloride, a highly effective, persistent, insecticide.

- **Ganglion** This may be defined as a nerve tissue where a number of nerve cells bodies are aggregated.

- **Gangrene** Invasion and putrefaction of necrotic tissue by saprophytic bacteria.

- **Gangrenous dermatitis** A disease of poultry, often associated with Infectious Bursal Disease and Inclusion-Body, Hepatitis.

- **Gap** An unoccupied interval in time.

- **Garget milk** Milk drawn from an animal suffering from an acute form of mastitis.

- **Gas Gangrene** is an acute bacterial disease due to the inoculation of wounds with organisms belong to the 'gas gangrene' group.

- **Gastr(o)** Stomach.

- **Gastralgia** Pain in the stomach.

■ **Gastrectomy** is an operation for the removal of the whole or part of the stomach.

■ **Gastric Dyspepsia** Abomasum become impacted.

■ **Gastric juice** A clear liquid secreted by the wall of the stomach. It contains hydrochloric acid and the enzymes rennin, pepsin and gastric lipase.

■ **Gastritis** Inflammation of stomach.

■ **Gastro-enteritis** Inflammation of both stomach and intestines.

■ **Gastrovascular** Serving for both digestion and circulation.

■ **Gaunt** A decrease in abdominal size.

■ **Gelatin** An organic colloidal substance made from animal bones, skins or hide fragments *or* A protein prepared by boiling collagen with water; used as a stabilizer in ice cream.

■ **Gene** The unit of inheritance, which is transmitted in the gametes or reproductive cells, and which by interaction with other genes and with the environment, controls the development of a characteristic.

■ **General** Usual, ordinary, vague.

■ **General anesthesia** It means a loss of sensation of the whole body.

■ **General Bacteriology** It is the study of the general characteristics of all bacteria.

■ **Generation interval** The average age of the parents when their offspring are born. Cattle-5 years; sheep-4 years; swine—2 ½ years.

■ **Genetic correlation** A condition where two or more quantitative traits are determined by many of the same genes.

■ **Genetic engineering** The replacement of a gene (usually defective) by a gene from an outside source i.e. introduction of a gene from one bacteria into another.

■ **Genetic value** The total value of all the genes an individual possesses for performance, type, or carcass quality and quantity.

■ **Genetics** Is the branch of biological science which seeks to account for the similarities and differences which are exhibited by related individuals, or simply the study of inherent similarities and differences.

■ **Genital system** System related acts with reproduction i.e. male genital system, female genital system.

■ **Genome** The total genetic composition of an individual or population inherited with the chromosomes.

■ **Genotype** The actual genetic makeup of an individual or population inherited with the chromosomes.

■ **Gentian violet** A stain used in microscopical work and a valuable antiseptic, of use against fungous and bacterial skin infections.

■ **Genus** is a group of species.

■ **Gerber test** for fat A test for determining fat in milk.

■ **Germ** Living substance capable of developing into an organ, part, or organism as a whole.

■ **Germ plasm** Genetic material in the form of sperm or ovum.

■ **Germicidal** Capable of killing microorganisms.

■ **Gerontology** Scientific study of the problem of ageing in all its aspects.

■ **Gestation** Pregnancy; in cows the period during which the unborn calf is carried in the uterus or womb of the mother.

■ **Gestational heat** When pregnant animal shows sign of heat.

■ **Giardia** A genus of flagellate protozoa.

■ **Gid** Disease in sheep caused by *Coenuras cerebralis*, an intermediate stage of *Taenia multiceps* of dogs.

■ **Gilt** A female pig intended for breeding purposes upto the time she has her first litter.

■ **Ginger** Dried rhizome of the tropical plant *Zingiber officinale*.

■ **Gingiva** Means gums.

■ **Gingivitis** Inflammation of gums

■ **Girdle** Skeletal structures of vertebrates by which the appendages are associated with the trunk.

■ **Gizzard** Stomach of poultry.

■ **Glanders** Glanders is a contagious disease characterized by nodules or ulcers in the respiratory tract and on the skin in any affected horse population is caused by *Malleomyces mallei*.

■ **Glands** A term loosely applied to a number of different organs. In each there are epithelial cells which have a secretory function.

■ **Gleet** A thin morbid discharge as from a wound.

■ **Glioma** is a tumour which forms in the brain or spinal cord.

■ **Gliosis** Proliferation of astrocytes in nervous tissue.

■ **Globulin** is a protein fraction of the blood plasma, associated with immunity.

■ **Glomerulonephritis** Nephritis involving primarily the glomeruli and extending secondarily into the surrounding interstitial tissue.

■ **Glomerulus** Small bunch of capillaries covered by thin epithelium, which projects into Bowman's capsule in kidney.

■ **Glossitis** Inflammation of tongue.

■ **Glottis** The opening from the pharynx into the larynx.

■ **Glouble** Small spherical particles, specially that of milk fat.

■ **Glucocorticoids** Refer to steroid hormones of the adrenal cortex.

■ **Gluconeogenesis** Formation of glucose from protein or fat.

■ **Glucose** Also known as dextrose. A simple six-carbon sugar (hexose) $C_6H_{12}O_6$, which is found naturally in plant tissues and formed by the hydrolysis of starch.

■ **Glutamic acid** is an amino acid.

■ **Gluteal** is the scientific name applied to the region of the buttocks.

■ **Glutin** the protein of wheat and other grains.

■ **Glutinous** Adhesive or sticky.

■ **Glutitis** Inflammation of gluteal muscles.

■ **Glycerin or Glycerol** is a clear, colourless, odourless, thick liquid of a sweet taste, obtained by decomposition and distillation of fats.

■ **Glycerophosphates** are compounds of glycerin with the respective phosphates. They are supposed to be specially useful for debility following a serious or wasting disease.

■ **Glycogen** A polysaccharide with the formula $(C_6H_{10}O_5)_n$ which is formed in the liver and muscle and depolymerised to glucose to serve as a ready source of energy when needed by the animal.

- **Glycogenesis** Conversion of glucose into glycogen.

- **Glycogenolysis** Conversion of glycogen into glucose.

- **Glycolysis** Conversion of carbohydrate into lactate by a series of catalysts. The breaking down of sugars into simpler-compounds.

- **Glycosides** Glycosides are ether-like, non-nitrogenous combinations of a sugar with other organic substances of glucoside is applied to those glycosides in which glucose is present. Glycosides may or may not contain nitrogen.

- **Glycosuria** presence of glucose in the urine

- **Goat** The goat, a small ruminant, belongs to the family Bovidae (hollow-horned ruminants) and is a member of the genus Capra.

- **Goiter** An enlargement of the thyroid gland located in the neck and is caused by an iodine deficiency.

- **Goitrogens** Refers to the substances which are found in foods and interfere with normal functioning of the thyroid gland and can cause goitre in animals.

- **Gonadotrophin** Hormones produced from gonads or reproductive organ.

- **Gonads** The primary sex glands which produce the reproductive cells or gametes, (testes in males', ovaries in the females).

- **Goshala** A charitable institution for keeping unwanted/culled cattle.

- **Gossypol** A substance present in cotton-seed and cotton-seed meal which is toxic to animals.

- **Gout** Deposition of calcium and sodium urates in connective tissue and serous membrane.

- **Graaffian follicle** See follicle.

- **Grade** An animal that is not a purebred but commonly showing characteristics of a particular breed. Usually one of their parents was purebred.

- **Grading up** Mating of a pure bred sire of a superior breed to non-descript cows.

- **Gram-negative** Bacteria which stain red with gram's stain.

- **Gram-positive** Bacteria which stain blue with gram's stain.

- **Granulocytosis** Presence of increased number of granulocytes in the blood.
- **Granuloma** A granular tumour.
- **Graph** Diagram or curve representing varying relationships between sets of data. Often used a word ending denoting a recording instrument.
- **Grass** Herbage suitable for grazing animals.
- **Grass** Tetany Magnesium deficiency in cattle. Lactation tetany.
- **Gravid** Pregnant.
- **Graze** Feed on growing grass.
- **Grease** which is also called *Seborrhoea* and *Stearrhoea*, is a form of chronic inflammation of the skin of the region of the fetlocks and pasterns of horses' legs.
- **Grey matter** Tissue of vertebrate central nervous system containing numerous cell-bodies and dendrites of nerve cells.
- **Grinding** Grinding is that process by which a feedstuff is reduced to a particle size by impact, shearing or attrition.
- **Groat** Grain from which the hulls has been removed.
- **Grooming** Term used in connection with animals that comprises cleaning, brushing, and combing etc. of the animal's body coat.
- **Groundnut oil cake** The oil-cake obtained after the mechanical extraction of oil from decorticated groundnut kernels.
- **Growth** Increase in size and dry-weight of an organism or cell.
- **Growth hormone** Hormone secreted by anterior pituitary. It stimulates growth by its action on carbohydrate and protein metabolism.
- **Gruel** A thin paste or thick fluid of oatmeal or maize meal, milk and water.
- **Grunting** It is a forced expiration against a closed glottis which happens in many types of painful and laboured breathing.
- **Gynaecological** Pertaining to gynaecology.
- **Gynaecology** Study of female reproduction including its diseases.

❏

H/h

■ **Habitat** The natural abode of an animal or plant.

■ **Habitual** Customary, routine, usual.

■ **Haematology** Study of blood, its constitutents and the diseases connected with it.

■ **Haematoma** is a swelling containing blood. It is found upon parts of the surface of the body.

■ **Haematometra** A collection of blood and other menstrual fluid within the uterus which causes the uterus to distend (bulge outward).

■ **Haematuria** Presence of blood in the urine

■ **Haemochorial placenta** A type of placenta where the chorion, or membrane enclosing the foetus, comes in direct contact with the mother's blood. Humans have haemochorial placentas.

■ **Haemoendothelial placenta** A haemoendothelial placenta is a type of placenta in which the inner lining (endothelium) of the capillaries of the chorion (membrane enclosing the foetus) comes in direct contact with the mother's blood.

■ **Haemoglobin** A pigment present in the erythrocytes.

■ **Haemoglobinuria** The presence of haemoglobin in the urine.

■ **Haemolysis** The destruction of red blood corpuscles and the consequent escape from them of haemoglobin.

■ **Haemobartonella** microorganism of the family bartonellaceae.

■ **Haemonchosis** Parasitic disease of sheep, goat and cattle caused by *Haemonchus sp.*

■ **Haemophilia** is a disease which the affected animal bleeds upon the slightest provocation, and in which the haemorrhage is very difficult to control.

■ **Haemopoiesis** Formation of blood.

■ **Haemorrhage** Escape of all constituents of blood from any part of vascular system.

■ **Haemorrhagic septicaemia** The bacterial disease commonly called '*gul ghottu*' is an acute septicaemia caused by *Pasteurella multocida.*

- **Haemostatics** are means taken to check bleeding, and may be either drugs applied to the area, or mechanical devices, etc.

- **Haemothorax** Accumulation of whole blood in the thoracic cavity.

- **Hairballs** Round objects consisting of hair land other food particle.

- **Half-sibs** Half brothers and half-sisters. The Individual having one common parent either mother or father.

- **Hallucination** A sense perception that has no basis in external stimulation.

- **Haloxon** An organo-phosphorus compound used against gastro-intestinal nematode worms.

- **Hamburger** Ground beef prepared from the less tender cuts.

- **Hammer** Instrument with a head designed for striking blows.

- **Hamster** Small rodent used extensively in laboratory experiments.

- **Hard paid disease** Syn. canine distemper.

- **Hatchery** The place where fertilized eggs are kept in incubators for a specific period of time till a day old chick emerges.

- **Hay** Forage preserved in dry form without any appreciable loss in its nutritive value.

- **Haylage** Haylage is a low moisture silage (40 to 45 per cent moisture) and is made from grass/or legume that is wilted to 40–45 per cent moisture content before ensiling.

- **HDL** High-density lipoproteins.

- **Healing** It is a process in which the body destroys and removes the irritant or returns the part to as near as normal functional state as possible.

- **Healing** powders Nonirritant powders are employed as vehicles for the incorporation of added medicinal agents.

- **Health** It is the state of an individual living in complete harmony with his environment.

- **Healthy** Hale, sound, robust, lusty.

- **Heart** It is a hollow muscular organ consisting of two atria, the receiving chambers and two ventricles,—the discharging chambers, which acts as a central pump for pulmonary and systemic circulation.

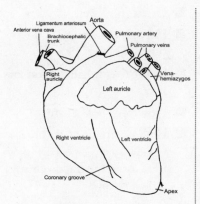

HEART OF COW

■ **Heart worms** *Dirofilaria immitis* is a common parasites of dogs. This infestation is known as canine filariasis or Dirofilariasis.

■ **Heat** Sexual excitement.

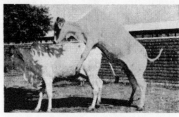

HEAT IN COW

■ **Heat increment** The heat which is unavoidably produced by an animal incidental with nutrient digestion and utilization was originally called work of digestion.

■ **Heat stability of milk** The time required to ensure coagulation in milk.

■ **Heat-stroke** is a condition associated with excessively hot weather, and, especially under conditions of stress. *Symptoms* The animal great lethargy and inability for work or movement, temperature very high. Death often takes place in a few hours.

■ **Hecto**—word element—hundred ; used in units of measurements.

■ **Heifer** Young cow that has never had a calf.

■ **Heliotherapy** Therapeutic use of the sun bath.

■ **Helium** Chemical element.

■ **Helminthiasis** Worm infestation.

■ **Hemat (o)** Blood.

■ **Hematic** Pertaining to or containing blood.

■ **Hematocele** Accumulation of blood in the tunica vaginalis.

■ **Hematologist** Specialist in hematology.

■ **Hematology** Science dealing with morphology of blood and blood-forming tissues with their physiology and pathology.

■ **Hemi** Half.

■ **Hemisphere** Half of a spherical or roughly spherical structure or organ.

■ **Hemo** Blood.

■ **Hemocytometer** Instrument for counting the number of blod cells.

■ **Hemoglobinometer** Instrument for determining the percentage of hemoglobin in the blood.

■ **Hemolytic anemia** Anaemia which results from the hemolysis of red blood cells.

■ **Hemophilia** An inherited condition in which the blood does not clot normally.

■ **Hemostat** A small surgical clamp for constricting blood vessels.

■ **Hen Day Production** This is ascertained by dividing the total eggs laid by a flock in a day by a number of birds in the shed. This is expressed in percentage (%).

■ **Hen House Average** Total number of eggs laid by a flock in the entire laying period divided by the number of birds housed in the shed at the onset of laying.

■ **Heparin** Substance which prevents blood clotting by stopping conversion of prothrombin to thrombin

■ **Hepat (o)** Liver.

■ **Hepatic functions** Liver functions

■ **Hepatitis** Inflammation of liver.

■ **Hepatosis** See hepatitis.

■ **Herb** Leafy plant without a woody stem, especially one used as a household remedy or as a flavour.

■ **Herbage** Green plants collectively; specially those used for pasturage.

■ **Herbivorous** Subsisting upon plants.

■ **Herd** A group of cattle.

■ **Herdmates** Individuals within the same herd which do not have the same sire but their records are made under similar environmental condition and at approximately the same time.

■ **Hereditary** Physical and productive characteristics inherited from parents.

■ **Heritability** Phenotypic variation that is due to inheritance.

■ **Heritability estimate** An estimate of the proportion of the total phenotypic variation in a population that is due to heredity.

■ **Hermaphrodite** An individual having both ovarian and testicular tissue either united for as separate structures. (with both sexes)

■ **Hernia** Protrusion of abdominal viscera through a natural or artificial opening.

■ **Heterogametic** ; This term is often used in reference to the sex cells. Hetero means unequal or unlike.

■ **Heterotrophic** Those organisms which require an organic source of carbon for their growth are called heterotrophic.

■ **Heterozygote** An individual which contains two different phases (or allels) of a gene at corresponding locations on homologous (or paired) chromosomes.

■ **Hex** (a) Six.

■ **Hexachlorophen** A drug used against liver fluke.

■ **Hexamine** is a substance made by the action of amonia upon formalin.

■ **Hexamitiasis** Used for urinary infection.

■ **Hexapod** A six-footed animal; a true insect.

■ **Hibernation** The dormant state in which certain animals pass the winter, marked by narcosis.

■ **Hiccough** Sudden jerky expression of breath.

■ **High** temperature, short time (HTST) pasteurization Milk is heated to a temperature of 71°C to 72°C for not less than 15 seconds and immediately cooled to below 10°C.

■ **Hinny** The offspring of a jennet, or female ass, and a stallion. It is the reciprocal of the mule.

■ **Hip Bones** Each hip bone consists of three large flat bones-Ilium, Ischium and Pubis.

■ **Hip joint** Ball and socket. Cotyloid cavity of os coxae and head of femur.

■ **Hist** Tissue.

■ **Histamine** Histamine is present in by basophils/mast cells and is released following injury. It causes vasodilation, increased vascular permeability and induces pain.

■ **Histidine** One of the essential amino acids.

■ **Histology** Department of anatomy dealing with

the minute structure, composition and function of tissue.

■ **Histology** Study of fine structure of an organism with the use of microscope.

■ **Hock joint** Distal end of tibia, tarsal bones, Lateral and proximal ends of metatarsal bone.

■ **Hog** A male pig after being castrated.

■ **Hog cholera** Swine fever.

■ **Hogget** One-year-old sheep.

■ **Hol (o)**—Word element; Entire, whole.

■ **Homeo** Similar; same; unchanging.

■ **Homeopathy** A system of therapeutics based on the administration of minute doses of drugs which are capable of producing in healthy persons symptoms like those of the disease treated.

■ **Homeostasis** Maintenance of body fluids (as opposed to fluid within cells) at the correct pH and chemical composition.

■ **Homo** Same.

■ **Homodont** Having all the teeth of the same kind in most vertebrates, other than mammals.

■ **Homogenizer** A device to break up cells/tissues so as to make the particles uniformly small and evenly distributed.

■ **Homogenous** of uniform quality, composition.

■ **Homologous chromosomes** The Chromosomes occur in body cells in pairs, one member of each pair having come from the sire and the other from the dam. The two members of a pair are spoken of as homologous chromosomes.

■ **Homozygote** An individual which possesses like genes in a pair found in body cells. For example, BB and bb individuals are said to be homozygous.

■ **Honey** Sweet-tasting substance produced by the honeybee.

■ **Hoof** Hooves are the hard and horny coverings of the ends of the digits. Hoof comprises of three parts— Periople, Wall and Sole.

■ **Hook** Curved instrument for traction holding.

■ **Hookworms** Small worms which attach themselves to the lining of the small intestine.

- **Hormone** An organic substance specifically produced by ductless glands (released directly into the bloodstream) to modify the rate of activity of another tissue.

- **Horns** The cornual processes of the frontal bones are enclosed by a horny covering. The horns as a whole form various curvatures and shape.

- **Hortvet apparatus** The apparatus used for determining freezing point of milk.

- **Hospital** An institute for the treatment of the sick.

- **Hot-air sterilization** Sterilization by the use fo an oven at 170°C for approximately 2 hours.

- **Hulls** The outer covering of threshed oats, rice etc.

- **Hum** A low, steady, prolonged sound.

- **Humerus** It is a long bone situated obliquely downward and backward, forms shoulder joint above with the scapula and elbow joint below with radius and ulna.

- **Humour** Any fluid or semi-fluid of the body.

- **Humus** Organic matter that remains in soil following partial decomposition.

- **Hunger** A purely local subjective sensation arising from gastric hypermotility caused in most cases by lack of distension by food.

- **Hyal (o)** Glassy.

- **Hyaline** A glassy or transparent substance or surface.

- **Hyaline degeneration** Accumulation of homogenous translucent substance in the tissue.

- **Hybrid** The offspring of two related individuals of the same species.

- **Hydrammas** Excessive accumulation of amniotic fluid in amniotic cavity.

- **Hydraulic process** A process for the mechanical extraction of oil from seeds, involving the use of a hydraulic press.

- **Hydroallantois** Excess accumulation of allanteic fluid in alantoic cavity.

- **Hydrocele** means a collection of fluid present within the outer proper coat of the testicle (tunica vaginalis) or within the spermatic cord.

- **Hydrocephalus** A condition in which there is excessive accumulation of cerebraespinal fluid in the cranial cavity.

■ **Hydrochloric acid** is normally present in the gastric juice. In the concenrated form it is like all other mineral acids, a corrosive and irritant poison.

■ **Hydrogen peroxide** An antimicrobial agent; can be used as milk preservative.

■ **Hydrogenation** The chemical addition of hydrogen to any unsaturated compound.

■ **Hydrolysis** The splitting of a substance into the smaller units by its chemical reaction with water.

■ **Hydrometer** An instrument for determining the specific gravity of a fluid.

■ **Hydrometra** Accumulation of watery fluid in the uterus.

■ **Hydronephrosis** Dilatation of renal pelvis due to obstruction of free flow of urine.

■ **Hydropericardium** Prese-nce of fluid in the pericardial sac.

■ **Hydrophobia** Disliking for water (As in Rabies).

■ **Hydropic degeneration** The disturbance of protein metabolism in which cell swells due to the presence of clear fluid.

■ **Hydrosalpinx** Cystic dilatation of fallopian tube due to clear fluid.

■ **Hydrotherapy** Use of water in any form in the treatment of disease.

■ **Hydrothorax** Accumulation of oedematous fluid in the pleural sacs.

■ **Hygiene** means the study of the various methods that should be taken to conserve the health, and to prevent preventable diseases.

■ **Hygroma** is a swelling occurring in connection with a joint, usually the knee or hock.

■ **Hygromycin B** An antibiotic used as an anthelmintic and claimed to be effective against large roundworms and whipworms.

■ **Hygroscopic** Readily absorbing water.

■ **Hyostrongylus rubidus** Parasitic worm of pigs.

■ **Hyper** A prefix which means above, beyond, or excessive.

■ **Hyperaemia** means congestion, or the presence of an excessive amount of blood in a part.

■ **Hyperaesthesia** It means oversensitiveness of bright light, sudden noise or touch.

■ **Hyperchromic** A significant increase in mean corpuscular hemoglobin. It is not known to occur. It is recommended that this term be avoided.

■ **Hyperimmunization** Repeated injections of large amounts of an antigen producing the maximum antibody response.

■ **Hyperkeratosis** Thickening of stratum corneum due to increased number of keratinized cells.

■ **Hypermotility** Increased movement.

■ **Hyperorexia** Increased appetite due to increased hunger contractions.

■ **Hyperpnoea** is defined as increased pulmonary ventilation.

■ **Hypersensitivity** Refers to a specifically induced hyperreactivity and is used synonymously with allergy.

■ **Hypertension** An abnormally high tension—usually associated with high blood pressure.

■ **Hyperthermia** Simple elevation of the temperature without systemic disturbances.

■ **Hyperthyroidism** Overactivity of the thyroid gland.

■ **Hypertonic** A solution of higher osmotic pressure than another solution to which it is compared (isotonic).

■ **Hypertrophy** means extra size or development of an organ or tissue.

■ **Hypervitaminosis** Disease associated with an excess of a particular vitamin.

■ **Hypnotics** Hypnotics are drugs used to depress moderately the central nervous systems of animals so that they are less responsive to stimuli.

■ **Hypo**—is a prefix indicating a deficiency.

■ **Hypochlorites** These are the longest known and probably most used chemical disinfectants.

■ **Hypochromic** Erythrocytes having mean corpuscular haemoglobin concentration below the mean normal values.

■ **Hypodermic** Applied or administered beneath the skin.

■ **Hypodermic Inj.** Administration of a solution through a fine, hollow needle into the tissues.

- **Hypogalactia** Reduction of milk production from udder due to infection etc.

- **Hypoglycaemia** is a deficiency of sugar in the blood.

- **Hypomagnesaemia** A condition in which there is too little magnesium in the bloodstream.

- **Hypomenorrhoea** A medical condition where the monthly menstruation period is abnormally short or where blood flow during menstruation is abnormally low.

- **Hypomotility** Reduced movement.

- **Hypophosphataemia** A condition in which the level of blood phosphorus is low.

- **Hypophysectomy** Surgical removal of pituitary gland.

- **Hypoplastic and aplastic anemia** Partial or complete suppression of blood cell production by the bone marrow.

- **Hypotension** Low arterial blood-pressure.

- **Hypotensive drugs** are used to produce temporary hypotensive in order to diminish haemorrhage.

- **Hypothalamus** A part of the brain below the thalamus which acts as a thermostat.

- **Hypothermia** Subnormal body temperature.

- **Hypogenesis** Defective embryonic development.

- **Hypoglossal** Beneath the tongue.

- **Hypoxia** Reduction of oxygen in the body tissues below level.

- **Hypothesis** to explain a group of phenomena and is assumed as a basis of reasoning and experimentation.

- **Hyster (o)** Uterus.

- **Hysterectomy** A surgical operation for removal of the uterus.

- **Hysteria (canine)** Young dogs which appear to be normal in every way are liable to attack so soon as they are subjected to any degree of exertion or excitement. The dog suddenly appears to 'go mad'. It races around with a fixed stare in its eyes, yelling or howling.

❑

I/i

- **I.L.T.** Infectious Laryngo-Tracheitis of fowls—caused by a virus.
- **I.Q.** Intelligence quotient.
- **I.U.** International unit or weighing unit.
- **Ice** cream A frozen dairy product made by suitable blending and processing of cream and other milk products, together with sugar and flavour.
- **Ichthyosis** A congenital skin disease in which epidermis continuously flakes off in large scale.
- **Icteric Index** It is a measurement of jaundice by comparing plasma colour with standard solution of potassium dichromate commonly used to know degree of jaundice.
- **Icterus / jaundice** A condition in which there is an excessive amount of haem-bilirubin or cholebilirubin or both causing them to become yellow.
- **ICU** Intensive Care Unit.
- **Idea** A mental impression or conception.
- **Idiosyncrasy** means a peculiarity of constitution causing an animal to react differently from most animals to a drug or treatment.
- **IgA** is an antibody/immuniglobulin found in the blood serum and also in secretion from mucous membranes. IgG and IgM are other immunoglobulins.
- **Ileitis** Inflammation of the ileum.
- **Ileum** It is the terminal part of small intestine and a thick tube. It is attached with cecum.
- **Ileus** Intestinal tympany.
- **Iliac** Relating to the flank.
- **Ilium** A pair of bones forming the sides of the birth canal as well as the "hooks" or hips.
- **Illness** A condition marked by pronounced deviation from the normal healthy state; sickness.
- **Imbalance** A term used to describe, for example, a faulty calcium-phosphorus ratio in the food of an animal; or an excess of one hormone in the blood stream.

■ **Imidazoles** Antifungal drugs that interfere with sterol synthesis.

■ **Immature** not fully developed; unripe.

■ **Immersion** The plunging of a body into a liquid.

■ **Immiscible** Not susceptible of being mixed.

■ **Immobilize** To render incapable of being moved.

■ **Immune** Possessing the capacity to resist infection.

■ **Immune bodies** Antibodies.

■ **Immune suppression** Suppression of antibody production.

■ **Immunity** An intrinsic or acquired state of resistance to an infectious agent.

■ **Immunization** The process of artificially producing resistance to a given infection generally by means of a vaccine.

■ **Immunology** The study of a host's specific defenses to a pathogen.

■ **Immunosuppression** Inhibition of the immune response.

■ **Immunotherapy** Treatment using antibodies.

■ **Immunotoxin** An immunotherapeutic agent consisting of a poison bound to a monoclonal antibody.

■ **Impaction** Sub-acute abdominal pain followed by one of acute pain. It can be due to acute intestinal obstruction with constipation.

■ **Impetigo** Impetigo is a superficial eruption of thin-walled, usually small, vesicle surrounded by a zone of erythema.

■ **Implantation** Adhering of the fertilized ovum to the uterine wall.

■ **Impotence** Complete failure of sexual power particularly in male.

■ **Impulse** The electrochemical process involved in neuro transmission of information and stimuli through out the body.

■ **In vitro** Something within an artificial environment, most likely within a glass tube.

■ **In vitro fertilization** Fertilization outside the body in a laboratory, the term test tube baby is inaccurate since fertilization occurs in a small circular dish, not a test tube.

■ **In vivo** Within the living body.

■ **Inanition** (**Malnutrition**) The diet is insufficient in quantity and all essential nutrients are present but in sub-optimal amounts.

■ **Inbreeding** A system of mating in which mates are genetically closely related than the average relationship. I.e., brother-sister, parent-offspring.

■ **Incarceration** Trapping of intestine internally from pressure on its external surface.

■ **Incidence** The rate at which a certain event occurs, as the number of new cases of a specific disease, occurring during a certain period.

■ **Incision** A cut or a wound made by cutting with a sharp instrument.

■ **Incisor** Adapted for cutting.

■ **Incisors** The incisors are most anterior in position and on either side are canines (teeth).

■ **Inclusion bodies** Small microscopic forms seen inside the cytoplasm or nucleus of a cell, in virus infections.

■ **Incompetent** Unable to function properly.

■ **Inco-ordination** is a term meaning irregularity in movement.

■ **Incubation** The growing of a culture of bacteria in an incubator to favour development of the organism.

■ **Incubator** An apparatus for maintaining cultures of bacteria and other materials at a constant and suitable temperature.

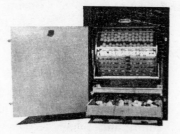

INCUBATOR

■ **Indicanuria** Presence of indican (potassium indoxyl sulphonate) in excessive amounts in urine.

■ **Indicator** A substance used in chemistry, to show by a colour change that a reaction has taken place.

■ **Indigestion** Indigestion is caused by atony of the forestomachs and is characterized clinically by anorexia, lack of ruminal movement and constipation.

■ **Indigo** A blue dyeing material.

■ **Induction** The process or act of inducing, or causing to occur.

■ **Inert** Inactive.

■ **Infantophagia** The eating of young ones by the animals.

■ **Infection** The successful invasion, establishment and growth of microorganisms in the tissues of the host.

■ **Infectious** Bovine Rhinotracheitis (IBR) is a highly infectious disease of bovines caused by a virus characterized by fever, nasal and ocular discharges, abortion, a relatively short course and a high recovery rate.

■ **Infectious** Bronchitis (IB) An acute, contagious and rapidly spreading virus disease of poultry characterized by gasping, coughing and crackling breathing sound, watery discharge from the nose, sometimes with a swelling of the sinuses.

■ **Infectious bursal disease** A viral disease also known as avain nephrosis/ gumboro disease.

■ **Infectious Coryza** An acute infectious disease caused by *Haemophilus gallinarum*, affecting the nasal passages and sinuses.

■ **Infectious disease** Which is caused by a microorganism bacteria, virus or protozoa.

■ **Infectious** Laryngotrachetis (ILT) A disease usually affecting adult birds, caused by herpesvirus. Also called chicken flue.

■ **Inferior** Below

■ **Infertility** Failure to breed.

■ **Infest** To occupy and cause injury to either a plant or to soil, or stored products.

■ **Infestation** A term used in connection with parasites affecting animal body.

■ **Inflammation** Reaction of the tissues to any injury and swellings.

■ **Influenza** Scientifically, this term is now applied only to disease caused by a virus.

■ **Infra** Beneath

■ **Infundibulum** Funnel shaped structure, at the ovarian end of the oviduct.

■ **Infusion** As a mode of administration of drug into a

gland i.e. through the teat canal in the mammary gland.

■ **Ingesta** Items which are taken by mouth.

■ **Ingluvitis** Inflammation of crop. Ingredients Any of the feed items that a mixture is made of.

■ **Inguinal canal** This is an oblique passage through the abdominal wall gives passage to round ligament of uterus in female, spermatic cord in male.

■ **Inhalation** Material in the form of vapor or dust is inhaled into the deeper air passages.

■ **Inheritance** Acquisition of characters or traits by transmission from parent to the offspring.

■ **Injection** Refers to the introduction of a solution, or a suspension, of a substance (usually a drug) through a hypodermic needle into the body. Injury Hurt, damage or harm.

■ **Inlet** A means or route of entrance.

■ **Inoculate** To introduce microorganisms into a culture medium or host.

■ **Inoculation** Introduction of micro organisms, infective material, serum or other substances into the tissues of living organism or culture media.

■ **Inoculum** Material used for inoculation. Inorganic Not of organic origin.

■ **Insanity** Craziness or madness.

■ **Inorganic** Denoting of mineral as distinct from animal and vegetabnle origin.

■ **Inscription** Listing of the names and amounts of the drugs to be incorporated in the prescription.

■ **Insecticidal agents** Drug used to "knock down" and to kill insects immediately after contact.

■ **Inseminate** To implant male sperm into the genital tract of female, either naturally or artificially.

■ **Instantization** The process by which dried milk and milk products are made instantly soluble by solublization or rehydration.

■ **Insulin** is a hormone secreted by part of pancreas where it is produced by the cell-islets of Langerhans.

■ **Insufflation** Blowing of powder or vapour into a cavity.

■ **Intercostal** Between ribs.

■ **Interferon** A protein produced in animal cells as a defence against virus.

■ **Intermediate Host** Temporary host in which asexual development takes place.

■ **Intermittent** Marked by alternating periods of activity and inactivity.

■ **Intern** A medical graduate serving and residing in a hospital preparatory to being licensed to practice medicine.

■ **Internal ear** The main portion of the organ of hearing and situated within the petrous temporal bone.

■ **Internal parasites** Parasites which live within the body.

■ **Interstitial** is a term applied to cells of different tissue set amongst the active tissue cells of an organ.

■ **Interval** The space between two objects or parts, the lapse of time between two events.

■ **Interosseous** Between bones. Intervertebral Between vertebrae.

■ **Intestine** Intestine is a very long tube which begins at the pyloric end of stomach and terminates at the anus.

■ **Intoxication** A state of poisoning by the toxin of an organism.

■ **Intra** Word element, within.

■ **Intracardial** Injection of the material directly into the heart.

■ **Intracellular** Refers to substances within the cell.

■ **Intracervical insemination** The artificial insemination of sperm into the cervical canal.

■ **Intracranial** Injections are made directly into the cranium.

■ **Intracutaneous** The material is injected into the skin.

■ **Intracytoplasmic sperm** The direct injection of a single sperm into an egg.

■ **Intradermal Injection** Injection of small amounts of drugs into the layers of the skin.

■ **Intramammary** Drugs adminstered by intramammary infusion in the mammary glands.

■ **Intramedullary Injection** Injection of drugs into the

sternal bone marrow with a special type of puncture needle.

■ **Intra-membranous Ossification** Formation of flat bones without formation of cartilage.

■ **Intramuscular** The inoculum is injected into the body of large muscles, such as those in the neck and the gluteal region.

■ **Intraocular** Substances injected into cornea, or into the anterior chamber of eye.

■ **Intraperitoneal injection** The term used for an injection into the peritoneal cavity.

■ **Intrapleural Injection** Drug administration in pleural cavity.

■ **Intrapulmonary** Substances are injected into the lungs.

■ **Intraspinal** Injection of material directly into the spinal canal.

■ **Intrathecal injection** Injection into the cerebrospinal fluid of the subaranchnoid space.

■ **Intrathoracic** Injections into the thorax. Intratracheal Fluids are injected into the trachea.

■ **Intrauterine contraceptive** A contraceptive device that is placed within the uterus for the purpose of inhibiting conception.

■ **Intravenous** The material is injected directly into a vein.

■ **Intrinsic factor** A protein released by gastric glands, essential for the satisfactory absorption of the extrinsic factor Vit. B_{12}.

■ **Introvert** A person whose interests are turned inward upon himself.

■ **Intussusception** Telescoping of a portion of intestine into another.

■ **Invertebrate** An animal without a dorsal column of vertebrae.

■ **Involution** After expulsion of fetus during puerperium the genital organs return to their normal non pregnant state.

■ **Involve** Complicate, entangle.

■ **Iodides** are salts of iodine. Sodium iodide is used in the treatment of actinobacillosis.

■ **Iodine** is a non-metallic element which is found largely in seaweed. It is prepared in the form of a dark violet-brown scales.

■ **Iodised salt** Usually 1 part of iodide in 25,000–50,000 parts of salt.

■ **Ion** An atom or a group of atoms (molecules) carrying an electric charge, which may be positive or negative.

■ **Ionophore** A substance that has been forming channels through a lipid membrane, including cell membranes, thus allowing ions to traverse the membrane along their concentration gradient.

■ **Iontophoresis** Drugs which are poorly absorbed through the skin can be forced through the skin by means of an electric current of about 50 milliamperes which passes through the tissue to be affected.

■ **I.P.** Indian Pharmacopoeia

■ **Iris** The pigmented diaphragm directly in front of the lens of the eyes. Its muscles by contraction adjust size of the pupil.

■ **Iron** Iron is best known element for being an active part of hemoglobin in red blood cell.

■ **Irradiation** Exposure to X-rays, radioactive material, ultra-violet; or infra-red rays.

■ **Irrigation** Washing by a stream of water or other fluid.

■ **Irritable** Touchy.

■ **Irritant** Causing irritatin.

■ **Irritation** Action of a drug on the nourishment, growth, and morphology of the cell.

■ **Ischemia** Local anaemia.

■ **Ischium** It is roughly a quadrilateral plate of bone situated behind the pubis and forms most part of the pelvic floor. Iso From the Greek word meaning equal.

■ **Isolation** Keeping animals separated from the rest of the herd, usually done when animals are suspected of suffering from some infectious or contagious disease. Also, quarantine.

■ **Isotonic solution** A solution having the concentration of both solvent and solute equal to those in another solution to which it is compared.

■ **Isotope** A form of a chemical element in which the number of neutrons in the nucleus is different from the other forms of that element.

■ **Itching** Pruritus; an unpleasant cutaneous sensation, provoking the desire to scratch or rub the skin.

■ **Itis** A suffix added to the name of the organ to signify inflammation of the organ.

■ **IVF** In Vitro Fertilization.

❑

J/j

- **Jack** An uncastrated male donkey.

- **Jaggery** The coarse dark sugar which is made from the sap of the coconut palm; or raw sugar cane juice, used in India as sweetening agent—also known as gur.

- **Janet** A female mule.

- **Jaundice** Jaundice is a clinical sign which often arises in diseases of the liver and biliary system

- **Jaw** The upper jawbones are two in number and are firmly united to the other bones of the face. The lower jaw-or mandible—is composed of a single bone in horse, pig, dog, and cat.

- **Jejunum** The middle portion of the small intestine which extends from the duodenum to the ileum.

- **Jelly** A soft coherent substance.

- **Jenny** A female donkey (ass). Also called a jennet.

- **Jerk** A sudden reflex or involuntary movement.

- **Johne's Disease or Para tuberculosis** Johne's disease is a specific, infectious enteritis of cattle, sheep and goats. It is characterized by progressive emaciation, chronic diarrhoea with thickening and corrugation of the wall of the intestine.

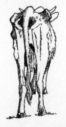

JOHNE'S DISEASE

- **Johnin** A diagnostic agent used for *Johne's* disease.

- **Joint** Place of union of two bones or other hard plates.

- **Joint ill** A disease in foals, when joints get inflamed and swollen.

- **Jugular** is the name of the large veins which carry the blood back to the chest from the head and anterior parts of the neck.

- **Juice** Any fluid from animal or plant tissue.

- **Junction** The place of meeting or coming together.

- **Junket** A simple form of soft rennet cheese, often made at home by curding milk with junket tablets, which contain rennet in dry form.

- **Jurisprudence** The science of law.

- **Juvenile** Pertaining to youth or childhood; young or immature.

- **Juxta** Near or adjoining to.

❏

■ **Kala-Azar or Dumdum fever** is a disease of human beings caused by a small protozoon parasite called the *Leishmania donovani.*

■ **Kanamycin** A broad-spectrum antibiotic derived from streptomyces kanamyceticus.

■ **Kaolin, or Chinese clay** is a native aluminium silicate, which is used as a protective and astringent dry dusting powder given internally is an adsorbent in intestinal disorders.

■ **Karyology** Study of structure of nucleus and function.

■ **Karyolysis** Lysis of the nucleus.

■ **Karyorhexis** Fragmentation of the nucleus.

■ **Karyoschisis** Appearance of cracks in the nucleus.

■ **Karyotype** The chromosomes of a plant or animal as they appear at the metaphase of a somatic division.

■ **Keel (Carina)** Thin platelike projection of bone from ventral surface of sternum of birds and bats, to either side of which powerful wing muscles are attached.

■ **Kefir** A self-carbonated beverage contaiing 1 per cent lactic acid and 1 per cent alcohol prepared by inoculating milk with kefir culture (grains).

■ **Keloid** Hypertrophic scar of the dermis following injury to skin.

■ **Kerat(o)** Intermediate Horney tissue..

■ **Keratin** A sulphur-containing protein which is the primary component of epidermis, hair, wool, hoof, horn, and the organic matrix of the teeth.

■ **Keratomalacia** Softening of the cornea caused by lack of Vit. A.

■ **Keratosis** Any horny growth, such as a wart, causing the cornification, or hardening, of the epithelial skin layers.

■ **Kernel** A dehulled seed.

■ **Ketonuria** Ketone bodies in urine.

- **Ketosis** (Acetonaemia) of ruminants
- **Ketosis** in ruminants is a disease caused by impaired metabolism of carbohydrates and volatile fatty acids, and is characterized by ketonaemia, ketonuria, hypo-gly caemia and low levels of hepatic glycogen.
- **Kidney** Organ of excretion of vertebrates. Nephrons are the blood filtering units of kidneys.
- **Kidneys** The kidneys are paired lobulated oval or bean shaped glands situated at the upper cranial part of the abdominal cavity and above peritonium.
- **Kilocalorie** (kC or kcal) The unit of heat used in nutrition. The amount of heat required to raise 100 g water 1°C (from 15.5 to 16.5 F); also known as the large calorie.
- **Kinetic** pertaining to or producing motion.
- **Kingdom** The highest category in the taxonomic hierachy of classification.

- **Kinins** Substances released from tissue cells that cause vasodilation.
- **Kjeldahl method for nitrogen estimation** A common method used for determination of nitrogen in milk and milk products.
- **Klebsiella** Microbe causing infection. Klebsiella infection may cause illness clinically.

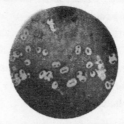

KLEBSIELA PNEUMONIA

- **Kumiss** A Russian fermented milk, mildly alcoholic.
- **Kuppfer cells** Fixed tissue macrophages lining the blood sinuses in the liver.
- **Kwashiorkor** A disease (syndrome) produced by a severe protein deficiency accompanied by characteristic changes in skin.

LD0 which is the maximum nonfatal dose, and LD100, which is the lowest lethal dose killing all animals.

LD50 The dose of drug fatal to 50 per cent of the animal is called the median lethal dose, or LD50.

L.H. (luteinizing hormone) Produced by the anterior pituitary and which assists in rupturing the Graffian follicle as well as stimulating the development of the corpus luteum.

Laceration The act of tearing.

Lachrymal glands Tear secreting glands.

Lactagogue Galactagogue.

Lactation The period following parturition (calving) during which the mammary glands secrete milk.

Lactation tetany Known as hypomagnesaemia.

Lactic Pertaining to milk.

Lactic acid An organic acid, one form ($CHOH$, CH_2, $COOH$) of which is commonly found in sour milk.

Lactogen (galactin) A hormone which brings about the secretion of a fluid resembling colostrum milk.

Lactoglobulin The fraction of milk serum proteins which is precipitated by 50 per cent saturation with ammonium sulphate. Colostrum contains much more lactoglobulin than normal milk.

Lactometer An instrument for measuring the specific gravity of milk.

Lactose Lactose of milk sugar is a disaccharide, composed of dextrose.

Lacuna a small pit or hollow cavity; gap.

Lamb Young sheep.

Lamb dysentery is an infectious ulcerative inflammation of the small and large intestine of young lambs, usually under 10 days old. Cause—*Clostridium welchii*.

Lambing Sheep giving birth to lamb.

Lameness consists of a departure from the normal

gait, occasioned by disease or injury situated in some part of the limbs or trunk and is usually accompanied by pain.

■ **Lamina** A thin, flat palate or layer.

■ **Laminated** Made up of laminae or thin layers.

■ **Laminitis** Inflammation of the sentitive laminae of the foot.

■ **Lamp** An apparatus for furnishing heat or light.

■ **Lampas** Inflammation of palate

■ **Lanolin** Purified, fatlike substance from the wool of sheep.

■ **Laparo** Flank; abdomen.

■ **Laparoscope** An endoscope for examining the peritoneal cavity.

■ **Laparotomy** means surgical opening of the abdominal cavity. The incision is either made in the middle line of the abdomen, or through one or other of the flanks.

■ **Lard** The fat rendered from fresh, clean, sound fatty tissues of hogs at the time of slaughter.

■ **Large intestine** The diameter of large intestine is greater at its first i.e. one and half meters and thereafter diminishes.

■ **Larva** Sexually immature stage of a helminth or arthropod.

■ **Laryngitis** Inflammation of the larynx. Laryngotomy Incision of the larynx.

■ **Larynx** An elongated musculo-cartilaginous compartment situated between the pharynx and trachea.

■ **Laser** A device that transfers light of various frequencies into an extremely intense small, and nearly non-divergent beam of monochromatic radiation in the visible region.

■ **Latent** Secret, inactive.

■ **Lavage** Gastric—the process of washing out the stomach.

■ **Lavish** Liberal, generous.

■ **Laxative** Refers to a substance that accelerates the passage of food through the intestine. If it alters peristalitic activity, it is termed a purgative; other types stimulate or depress the muscular activity of the gut.

■ **Leech** Annelids of the class Hirudinea, some species are bloodsuckers, and were formerly used for drawing blood.

■ **Leg** The lower limb, especially the part from knee to foot.

■ **Left atrium** It occupies the left caudal part of the base of the heart and is larger than the right atrium. It receives oxygenated blood.

■ **Left ventricle** The wall of this chamber is thickest of all the compartments of heart. It forms the left part of the heart.

■ **Legume** Refers to those crops that can absorb nitrogen directly from the atmosphere through bacteria that live in their roots. The clovers and alfalfa are common examples of legumes.

■ **Leishmaniasis** is the name applied to diseases of the blood caused by minute protozoan parasites.

■ **Leiomyoma** Benign uterine tumours also referred to as uterine fibroids.

■ **Length** an expression of the longest dimension of an object.

■ **Lens** Piece of glass or other transparent material so shaped as to converge or scatter light rays. Lens of eye of vertebrates, transparent structure just behind pupil, lying in aqueous humour, attached by collagen fibres to ciliary body.

■ **Leper** A person with leprosy.

■ **Leptocyte** A thin erythrocyte of decreased volume in relationship to its diameter often characterized by abnormality of shape.

■ **Leptomeningitis** Inflammation of inner and delicate membrane of brain and spinal cord.

■ **Leptospirosis** Infection with *Leptospira*.

■ **Lesbian** A female homosexual.

■ **Lesbianism** Homosexuality between women.

■ **Lesion** Macroscopic or microscopic alteration in tissue as a result of disease.

■ **Lethal gene** A gene which causes the death of an individual carrying it in the homozygous condition.

■ **Lethargy** A condition of drowsiness or indifference.

■ **Leucocytolysis** Destruction and disintegration of white blood cells.

■ **Leucocytosis** Increased number of leucocytes in the blood.

■ **Leucomalacia** Softening of white matter.

■ **Leucoma** The presence of an opaque patch spots on the surface of the cornea.

■ **Leucorrhoea** A pale yellowish discharge from the vulva.

■ **Leukemia** Neoplastic disease arising in haemopoietic tissue in which its type cells appear in the blood or are disseminated through the marrow. It is a form of cancer.

■ **Leukocytes (leucocytes)** The white cells of the peripheral blood stream.

■ **Leukoderma** Focal area of skin which lacks protein pigment.

■ **Leukopenia** Reduction of the number of leukocytes in the blood.

■ **Liberneck** In poultry—due to botulism.

■ **Libial** Pertaining to lips.

■ **Libido** Sexual desire or sex drive

■ **Lidocaine** A topical anesthetic.

■ **Life** The aggregate of vital phenomena; as metabolism, growth, reproduction, adaptation, etc.

■ **Ligament** A band of collagen connecting the two bones at a joint; helps restrict movement preventing dislocation.

■ **Ligate** To apply a ligature.

■ **Lignin** An indigestible compound which along with cellulose is a major component of the cell wall of certain plant materials such as wood, hulls, straws, and overripe hays.

■ **Limb** One of the paired appendages of the body used in locomotion.

■ **Lime** A corrosively alkaline earth, CaO.

■ **Limited feeding** Feeding animals to maintain weight and growth but not enough to fatten or increase production.

■ **Lincomycin** An antibiotic produced by Streptomyces lincolnensis.

■ **Line** A stripe, streak, mark, or narrow ridge.

■ **Line breeding** A system of breeding which involves the

mating of two animals to concentrate on the qualities of some superior ancestor.

■ **Linecross** An offspring produced by crossing two or more inbred lines

■ **Lingual** Pertaining to tongue.

■ **Liniments** These are liquid preparations of drugs dissolved or suspended in dilute alcohol or water

■ **Linkage** Two or more genes located on the same chromosome so that they tend to be transmitted together.

■ **Linked genes** Two or more genes that tend to be inherited together.

■ **Linoleic acid** An 18-carbon unsaturated fatty acid having two double bonds. It reacts with glycerol to form linolein. This is an essential fatty acid.

■ **Lipase** A fat-splitting enzyme.

■ **Lipids** A broad term for fats and fat-like substances.

■ **Lipoma** is a tumour mainly composed of fat.

■ **Lipotropic** Acting on fat metabolism by hastening removal or decreasing the deposit of fat in the liver.

■ **Lipolysis** The decomposition or splitting up of fat.

■ **Lipovaccine** A vaccine in a vegetable oil vehicle.

■ **Lips** are musculo-membraneous folds which act as curtains guarding the entrance to the mouth.

■ **Liquid** Soft clear fluid.

■ **Liquor** A liquid, especially an aqueous solution, or a solution not obtained by distillation.

■ **Listeriosis** Listeriosis is an infectious disease caused by *Listeria monocytogenes* and characterized by either meningoencephalitis, abortion or septicaemia.

■ **Litholapaxy** the crushing of a stone in the bladder and washing out of the fragments.

■ **Lithotomy** is the operation of opening the bladder for the removal of a stone.

■ **Lithotripsy** Litholapaxy.

■ **Litmus** A pigment prepared from Rocella tinctoria and other lichens; used as an acid-base (pH) indicator.

■ **Liver** The largest solid gland of the body. In fresh condition it is reddish brown in colour. It is placed in the right side of the abdominal cavity.

■ **Liver-flukes** are parasitic flat worms which infest the livers of various animals, especially sheep and cattle. They may cause illness and even death.

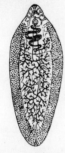

LIVER-FLUKES

■ **Liveweight** A term associated with the meat birds to indicate its weight before slaughter.

■ **Local anesthesia** It involves the loss of sensation of a limited area of the body.

■ **Lochial discharge** Discharge from uterus after parturition.

■ **Lock jaw** Tetanus in which the jaws become firmly locked together.

■ **Locomotion** Movement, or the ability to move, from one place to another.

■ **Locus** The region of a chromosome, or the pairs of homologous chromosomes where a particular gene is located.

■ **Logarithm (log)** Power to which a base number is raised to produce a given Fnumber. Logical Valid, sound, rational.

■ **Loins** The region of the lumbar vertebrae.

■ **Loose box** A single stable or pen for housing a single animal.

■ **Loose housing** Cattle yards and shelters large enough to permit cows to move at will from indoors to outdoors and from resting area to the place of feeding.

■ **Lotions** These are mild, liquid preparations for application to the skin without rubbing.

■ **LSD** Lysergic acid diethylamide. A psychedelic drug which produces behaviour and symptoms as hallucinations, delusions, etc.

■ **Lucerne** Leguminous fodder crop, perennial in nature and provides green nutritionally rich fodder throughout the year.

■ **Lugol's solution** A solution of 50 gm iodine and 100 gm potassium iodide in distilled water to 1000 cc.

■ **Lumbago** A form of rheumatism affecting the loins.

■ **Lumbar vertebrae** These vertebrae with their bodies form the bony roof of the abdomen.

■ **Lumber** Pertaining to abdominal region. Lumen Cavity of a tubular organ. Lungs Lungs are a pair of main organ of respiration. These are present in thoracic cavity.

■ **Lungworm** Any parasitic worm that invades the lungs.

■ **Luteinising hormone (L.H.)** This is the secretion or hormone of the anterior lobe of pituitary gland. L.H. controls the development of corpus luteum.

■ **Luteolytic agents** Agents that, in one way or another, are able to inhibit the corpus luteum's action to secrete progestogens.

■ **Luteolysis** Regression of the corpus luteum.

■ **Luxation** is another name for dislocation.

■ **Lymph** The slightly yellow, transparent fluid occupying the lymphatic channels of the body.

■ **Lymphangitis** The term lymphangitis denotes inflammation and enlargement of the lymph vessels.

■ **Lymphocyte** A type of white blood cell which has its origin in the lymph glands and is mononuclear.

■ **Lysine** is a very important amino acid to improve performance and to avoid using so much protein.

■ **Lysis** means the gradual ending of a fever, as opposed to 'crisia', which means the sudden termination of disease.

■ **Lyssa** Another name for rabies.

❑

- **Maceration** Softening of foetus and is associated with infection in the uterus.

- **Maconium** Brown or blackish, viscid, semifluid or hard material which collects in the bowels of young animals prior to birth.

- **Macrocyte** Large red blood cell found especially in association with a megaloblastic anemia.

- **Macrophage** A large mononuclear cell containing a spherical nucleus. In the circulating blood it is known as monocyte.

- **Macroscopic** Large enough to be visible to the naked eye.

- **Macula** Circumscribed flat discoloration of skin.

- **Mad** Insane, lunatic.

- **Mad** itch See pseudorabies.

- **Maedi** A chronic disease of sheep, caused by a virus, and characterised by pneumonia, dypsonea.

- **Maggots** Larvae of dipterous flies.

- **Magnesium** is a light white metal which burns in air with the production of a brilliant white flame. The salts of magnesium used as drugs are the oxide, carbonate, and sulphate.

- **Magnet** An object having polarity and capable of attracting iron.

- **Magnificent** Superb, majestic.

- **Maintain** Justify, defend

- **Maize bran** The bran, which essentially comprises the husk.

- **Maize Germ cake** The cake obtained after extraction of oil from maize germ.

- **Maize germ oil cake (meal)** Solvent extraction of oil of maize germ cake.

- **Maize gluten meal** The product is the dried residue from maize after the removal of the larger part of the starch and bran by the process employed in the wet milling manufacture of maize starch.

- **Maize grit** The fine to medium sized crushed maize grain with little or none of the bran or germ.

- **Makkhan** See butter.
- **Mal** Illness; disease.
- **Malacia** Softening of a part or tissue in disease, e.g. osteomalacia or softening of the bones.
- **Malathion** An organic phosphorus insecticide used for the control of external parasites in cattle.
- **Male** An individual of the sex that produces spermatozoa.
- **Male genital organs** Organs of male genital system. These are Testicle, Vas deferens, Urethra and Penis.
- **Mallein test** An allergic test like 'Tuberculin' for diagnosis of glanders in equines.
- **Malformation** Defective or abnormal formation; deformity.
- **Malignant** catarrhal fever of cattle or gangrenous coryza An infectious fever of cattle and buffaloes, in which there are acute inflammatory changes in the mucous membranes of the respiratory system.
- **Malnutrition** Actually a general term indicating a deficit, excess, or imbalance of one or more essential nutrients.
- **Malpractice** Improper ; unskillful and faulty medical or surgical treatment.
- **Malt sprouts** The product is obtained by removing the developing buds of malted barley and the mixing together with malt hulls or any other parts of malt.
- **Malta fever** or Meditarranean fever of man caused by *Brucella melitensis* which is closely allied to *Brucella abortus*.
- **Maltose** A disaccharide of two glucose units produced as a result of action of amylase on starch used as an additive to infant food.
- **Mammal** Any animal that gives milk to suckle its young.
- **Mammary gland** Udder or glands which secrete milk.
- **Mammary veins** Veins carrying blood away from the udder and found just under the skin on the abdomen barrel of the cattle.
- **Mammoplasty** The Plastic re-construction of the breast, either to augment or reduce its size.
- **Manchester** wasting disease A progressive wasting and

stiffness of joints caused by feeding of *Solanum malacoxylon.*

■ **Mandible** The lower jaw of vertebrates.

■ **Mange** Contagious skin disease caused by several species of mites which are transmitted by contact.

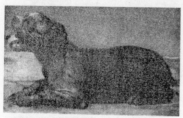

DEMODECTIC MANGE

■ **Manganese** is a metal of which the oxides are abundantly found in Nature.

■ **Manger** Feeding trough for animals.

■ **Monozygote** twin From one fertilized ovum due to its division two identical offspring develop.

■ **Marbling** The distribution of fat within the muscular tissue which gives the meat a white spotted appearance.

■ **Marine** Pertaining to or inhabiting the sea or other salt waters.

■ **Marek's Disease** Viral disease of poultry and affects the nervous system, various visceral organs, eyes, skin and muscles. Highly contagious. High rate of mortality.

■ **Market milk** Fluid milk sold to the consumers.

■ **Marrow** means the softer substance that is enclosed within the cavities of the bones.

■ **Masculine** Pertaining to the male sex.

■ **Mash** A type fo feeding method meant to supplement grain. It consists of a mixture of ground grains, grain by-products such as brans, middling, oilcake, minerals and animal by-products.

■ **Mask** To cover or conceal.

■ **Mass** A lump or collection of cohering particles.

■ **Mast cell** A type of cell found throughout the body that contains histamine and other substances that stimulate vasodilation.

■ **Mastication** Cutting of food into smallest possible pieces in the mouth by the animal.

- **Mastitis** Inflammation of mammary gland.

- **Masturbation** It refers to the self arousal of sexual responses in males.

- **Materia medica** An older term encompassing the entire field of pharmacy and pharmacology.

- **Metritis** Inflammation of uterus.

- **Maxilla** One of pair of large bones of the upper jaw of vertebrates in mammals.

- **Meal** A feed ingredient (meat, oat) having a particle size somewhat larger than flour.

- **Meatus** is a term applied to any passage or opening.

- **Mechanism** The manner of combination of parts, processes, etc., which serves a common function.

- **Meconium** The first faeces of the calf.

- **Median plane** Divides the body into two similar halves along the longitudinal axis.

- **Mediastinum** The right and left pleural sacs are separated from each other by an interpleural space at the midline—known as mediastinum.

- **Medical** pertaining to medicine.

- **Medicated** Imbued with a medicinal substance.

- **Medication** The administration of remedies.

- **Medicine** Any drug or remedy. The art and science of the diagnosis and treatment of disease and the maintenance of health.

- **Medical** Bacteriology The study of those bacteria, viruses, yeasts, and molds which are detrimental to the health of man and animals, primarily by their ability to produce disease.

- **Medium** In bacteriology this term is applied to a liquid (e.g. broth) or a solid which bacteria are grown in the laboratory.

- **Medulla (I)** The marrow in the centre of a long bone.

- **Medulla Oblongata** It is the cranial continuation of the spinal cord and extends from the foramen magnum to the caudal margin of pons.

- **Megacalorie** 1,000 kilocalories or 1,000,000 calories.

- **Mega** Megalo are prefixes denoting largeness.

■ **Megaloblast** A large, nucleated, primitive red blod cells.

■ **Melanin** The dark brown or black pigment seen in the hair and/or skin.

■ **Meiosis** A type of cell division responsible for producing the sex cells which normally posses the haploid number of chromosomes.

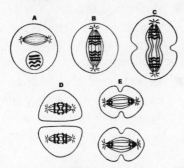

MEIOSIS OF CELL

■ **Menadione** Syn Vit. K.

■ **Menarche** The establishment or beginning of the menstrual function.

■ **Meninges** The brain and spinal cord are enclosed by three membranous coverings for their protection. These are known as meninges.

■ **Meningitis** Inflammation of the meninges.

■ **Menopause** The Cessation of the menstruation in the human female, occuring usually around the age of 50.

■ **Menthol** An alcohol from various mint oils ; used locally, to relieve itching.

■ **Meperidine** A narcotic analgesic.

■ **Mercurochrome** An antiseptic, and a stain for spermatozoa.

■ **Mercury** also known as quicksilver, and hydrargyrum, is a heavy silver-coloured liquid metal.

■ **Mesentery** is the double layer of peritoneum which supports the small intestine.

■ **Mesometrium** is the fold of peritoneum running from the roof of the abdomen to the uterus.

■ **Metabolic** Relating to metabolism.

■ **Metabolism** The sum total of the chemical changes in the body, including the building up (assimilation) and the breaking down (catabolic, dissimilation) process.

■ **Metabolite** Any substance produced by metabolism.

■ **Metabolizable** energy Digestible energy minus the energy of the urine and fermentation gases.

■ **Metacarpal Bones** There are two metacarpal bones. One is large and the other is small. Two fully developed digits (3rd and 4th) are present in the ox. Second and fifth digits are rudimentary. Each of the developed digits has three phalanges.

■ **Metacercaria** The encysted stage of a fluke in its final intermediate host.

■ **Metaphase** The second stage of mitosis in which the chromosomes are aligned on the equator of the spindle fibers.

■ **Metastasis** Spread of malignant cell from one part of the body to another by way of lymphatics or blood vessels as an embolus.

■ **Metatarsal bones** One large bone representing 3rd and 4th fused metatarsal and a small bone representing 2nd metatarsal.

■ **Meter (m)** the standard unit of length in the metric system; one ten-millionth of the distance from the equator to the pole.

■ **Methane** Odorless, colorless, flammable gas; CH_4.

■ **Methionine** One of the essential amino acids. It is sulphur containing and may be replaced in part by cystine.

■ **Methyl** is the name of an organic radicle whose chemical formulae is CH_3, and which forms the centre of a wide group of substances known as the methyl group.

■ **Methylated** spirit is a mixture of rectified spirit with 10 per cent by volume of wood naphtha.

■ **Methylene** blue given intravenously at a dose of 10 mg/kg of a 4 per cent solution, is an antidote to nitrate poisoning.

■ **Methyl red (MR) test** An indicator test for detecting the presence of acid products of fermentation.

■ **Methylene blue test** A test for determining freshness of milk.

■ **Metoestrus** is the period in the oestrous cycle following ovulation and during which the corpus luteum develops.

■ **Metrology** Metrology is the study of weights and measures used in prescription writing.

■ **Metrorrhagia** Uterine bleeding, usually of normal amount, occurring at completely irregular intervals.

■ **Micro** is a prefix meaning small.

■ **Micro ingredient** Any ration component normally measured in milligrams or micrograms per kilogram or in parts per million.

■ **Microaerophile** An organism that grows best in an environment with less oxygen (O_2) than is normally found in air.

■ **Microbe** A minute living entity, viral, bacterial, fungal or protozoan, too small to be seen without the aid of a microscope. Also called micro-organisms.

■ **Microbiology** Branch of biology dealing with the structure and function of microorganisms.

■ **Microcyte** An erythrocyte having a diameter below the normal range.

■ **Microflora** Microorganisms present in an organ/area e.g. fungi and bacteria of an area.

■ **Microgram** One-thousandth part of a milligram; symbol 'g'.

■ **Micrometer (m)** A unit of measure equal to 10–6m.

■ **Microphthalmia** An abnormal smallness of the eyes, accompnaied by blindness.

■ **Microscope** The ordinary microscope with oil-immersion lens gives magnification up to 1500 diameters.

■ **Microsporum** A group of fungi responsible for ringworm.

■ **Micron** One thousandth of a milimeter; a unit of microscopic measure.

■ **Microwave** An electromagnetic wave with wavelength between 10–1 and 10–3 m.

■ **Midcycle pain** One-sided lower abdominal (pelvic) pain that occurs at or around the time of ovulation (midcycle).

■ **Middle ear (tympanic cavity)** It is an irregularly biconcave small space within the petrous temporal bone.

■ **Miekev's nodule** Please see Pseudocowpox

■ **Migraine** A syndrome, the most common symptom of which has been periodic severe headache which has been vascular in origin an usually pulsative and unilateral in the initial phase.

- **Milbemycin** The term used for a family of macrolide antibiotics which kill insects and mites.

- **Milk** A white or yellowish fluid secreted by the mammary gland of mammals.

- **Milking** The pressing out of the contents of a tubular structure by running the finger along it.

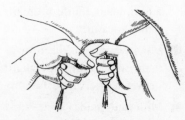

MILKING FULL HAND

- **Milk fat** Milk fat is composed of a number of glyceride esters of fatty acids, which are both saturated and unsaturated.

- **Milk fever** A metabolic disease occurring most commonly at the time of parturition and is characterized by muscular weakness, hypocalcaemia, circulatory collapse and depression of consciousness.

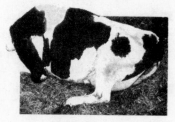

MILK FEVER

- **Milk ring** test for brucellosis, is a method of detecting infected herds of dairy cattle.

- **Milk yield** the average yield of dairy cows.

- **Milker's nodule** See Pseudocowpox

- **Miller's disease** *See* Bran disease.

- **Milk filter** A filter cloth or pad of the desired pore size which can retain the smallest particle.

- **Milk plasma** When fat is removed from milk, the part remaining is known as plasma.

- **Milk protein** Milk contains two different groups of proteins (a) the casein complex, present in the milk as a colloidal suspension; (ii) the whey proteins, present in the milk as a solution.

- **Milk sinus** Chamber situated at the base of the teats,

into which the milk tubules discharge their milk.

■ **Milk teeth** This is a temporary set of tooth and is replaced by permanent set.

■ **Milk well** Area on the body of cow where milk veins enter body cavity.

■ **Mineral salts** Refer to the inorganic salts, including sodium, potassium, calcium, chloride, phosphate, sulphate, etc.

■ **Mineral waters** The term used for the natural, untread, spring waters.

■ **Mineralisation** It is a general term for calcification/ossification/chondrification.

■ **Minerals** The term minerals in nutrition usually refers to inorganic ions in their elemental form (e.g., sodium, iodide, calcium).

■ **Miracidium** The free-swimming ciliated larva of a fluke that hatches from the egg.

■ **Miscarriage** Loss of the products of conception form the uterus before the fetus is viable; spontaneous abortion.

■ **Miscellaneous** Dissimilar, diversified.

■ **Mites** parasite associated with mange in all animals.

■ **Mithun** An obscure, shy, semi-wild bovine animal (*Bos frontalis*), confined to valleys in India

■ **Miticidal** Agent (s) which kill the mites.

■ **Mitosis** A cell division process in which the chromosomes are duplicated, followed by division of the cytoplasm of the cell.

■ **Mitotic centers** Two polarizing units of cell located opposite each other with spindle fibres at the proper stage of cell's division connecting them.

■ **Mixed culture** A culture containing more than one kind of microorganism.

■ **Mixed infection** Due to the presence of more than one species of organism.

■ **Mixtures** Mixtures are dispersions of insoluble solid substances in water, frequently with a stabilizing agent added.

■ **Mode** Refers to the most commonly occurring value in a series of measurements.

■ **MOET** Multiple Ovulation and Embryo Transfer.

■ **Molars** Permanent crushing back teeth of mammals which have no predecessors in the milk teeth.

■ **Molasses** A thick, viscous, usually dark coloured, liquid product containing a high concentration of soluble carbohydrates, minerals, and certain other material.

■ **Molds** All of the fungi that grow in a colony composed of loose threads are molds.

■ **Molecular biology** The science dealing with DNA and protein synthesis of living organisms.

■ **Molecular weight** The sum of the atomic weights of all atoms making up a molecule.

■ **Molting** The shedding of the hair, feathers, or outer layer of the skin, which are replaced by new growth.

■ **Molybdenum** This trace element is commonly present in soil and pasture grasses, and is beneficial.

■ **Monilia** A group of yeast-like organisms.

■ **Monoplegia** means paralysis of a single limb, or part.

■ **Monochid** A male animal which has only one testicle in the scrotum. Sometimes also called a ridgling.

■ **Monoclonal antibody** An extremely pure antibody derived from a single clone of an antibody-producing cell.

■ **Monohybrid** An individual heterozygous for a single pair of genes such as Aa.

■ **Monohybrid** cross A cross of two individuals involving a single pair of genes (alleles).

■ **Monster** Animal in which excessive abnormal development is present.

■ **Moraxella** Outbreaks of conjunctivitis and keratitis often associated with *M. bovis*.

■ **Morbid changes** Changes observed at necropsy that are as a result of disease.

■ **Morbidity** Percentage of exposed animals that get affected.

■ **Morphine** The main alkaloid of the opium poppy *Papaver somniferum* and the prototype narcotic analgesic drug.

■ **Morphology** The external appearance.

■ **Mortar** A bell—or urn-shaped vessel in which drugs

are beaten, or ground with a pestle.

■ **Mortality Rate** Mortality rate is expressed as the percentage of affected animals which die compared with total number of animals.

■ **Mosquito** a bloodsucking and venomous insect of the family culicidae.

■ **Motility** The ability of an organism to move by itself.

■ **Motor** Pertaining to muscles, movement and stimulation of effector organs.

■ **Moulting in poultry** When they stop laying eggs and go through a period of quiescence. Feathers may drop off.

■ **Mouth** It is bounded externally by lips and cheeks and internally by gums and teeth.

■ **Mucilage** is prepared from acacia or tragacanth gum, and is used as in ingredient of mixtures. It is also a demulcent.

■ **Mucolytics** Agents which soften mucous for expulsion.

■ **Mucopurulent** Containing a mixture of mucus and pus.

■ **Mucometra** Accumulation of viscid mucus like fluid in the uterus.

■ **Mucormycosis** Infectious condition of animals caused by fungi (*Mucor* sp.).

■ **Mucosa** Name given to the moist tissue lining. e.g., the mouth (buccal mucosa)—intestines and respiratory tract.

■ **Mucosal block** Self limiting absorption of iron as per requirement

■ **Mucous membrane** lines many hollow organs, the air passages, the whole of the alimentary canal and the ducts of glands urinary passages and genital passages.

■ **Mucus** is the slimy secretion derived from mucous membranes.

■ **Mulberry Heart Disease** Dietetic microangiopathy of pigs.

■ **Mule** The offspring of a male ass and a mare.

■ **Multiparous / palytocus** Those which give birth to more than two.

■ **Multiple alleles** A series of more than two alleles which occupy the same location on homologous chromosomes.

■ **Multiple factors** Two or more pairs of genes or factors that contribute to the expression of a chracteristic are called multiple factors.

■ **Mummification** Shrivelling of dead and retained foetus and is not associated with infection.

■ **Mumps** Swelling of face just below the ear,

■ **Muscular** relaxants are drugs, other than anaestheticfs, which produce relaxation or paralysis in voluntary muscle.

■ **Muscle** Tissue consisting of cells which are highly contractile. Responsible for movement.

■ **Mute** Unable to speak.

■ **Mutation** A permanent change in a gene which may result in a change in the phenotype of an individual.

■ **Mutualism** Association of two species as a mutually beneficial partnership.

■ **Muzzle** The region of the upper lip.

■ **Myalgia** means pain in a muscle.

■ **Mycology** The science dealing with fungi.

■ **Mycobacterium** One of a group of organisms which include the causes of tuberculosis and Johne's disease.

■ **Mycocardium** The heart muscle.

■ **Mycoplasma** An infective agent distinct from bacteria as well as from viruses.

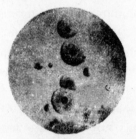

MYCOPLASMA

■ **Mycoplasmosis** A mycoplasma infection.

■ **Mycoplasma gallisepticum** It is responsible for CRD in poultry.

■ **Mycotoxin** A toxin produced by a fungus.

■ **Mycosis** are diseases due to the growth of fungi in the body.

■ **Mycotoxicosis** Poisoning by toxins produced by fungi.

■ **Mydriasis** means an unusual state of dilatation of the pupil of the eye.

- **Myelitis** Inflammation of the spinal cord.
- **Myelocyte** A bone-marrow cell, from which white cells of the blood are produced.
- **Myelomalacia** Softening of spinal cord.
- **Myiasis** Indicates the presence of larvae of dipterous flies in tissues and organs in a living animal.
- **Myocardial Asthenia** Myocardial asthenia or weakness is manifested by decreased power of contraction resulting in reduction of cardiac reserve.
- **Myocarditis** Inflammation of the heart muscle (Myocardium).
- **Myogen** Refers to the protein of muscle.
- **Myoglobinuria** Presence of myoglobin in the urine.
- **Myology** Study of muscles
- **Myometritis** Inflammation of muscular layer of uterus only.
- **Myopathy** The term myopathy describes the non-inflammatory degeneration of skeletal muscle characterized clinically by muscle weakness.
- **Myostitis** Inflammation of muscle.
- **Myosis** means an unusual narrowing of the pupil.
- **Myotics** are drugs which contract the pupil of the eye, such as eserine and opium

❏

Nagana is an unscientific but convenient name for trypanosomiasis transmitted by tsetse flies.

Nails or Claws are composed of modified skin substance which has become horny.

Nanometer (nm) A unit of measurement equal to $10^{-9}\,\mu m$, $10^{-3}\,\mu m$, or 10A.

Naphthol is a coal-tar derivative produced during the manufacture of coal gas.

Narcosis Stuporous state induced by a drug.

Narcotic Pertaining to or producing narcosis.

Narcotic drug Literally, a drug that produces nacrosis; i.e., reversible insensibility or stupor.

Nasal bot fly Larvae are serious parasites of sheep.

Nasal Cavity This is an elongated cavity enclosed by some facial bones and divided by a septum.

Nasal decongestant drug A drug that diminishes the resistance to airflow through the nose that accompaniest he common cold or hay fever.

Natal Pertaining to birth.

Natural Usual, regular, normal.

Natural immunity The immunity of an animal to disease or parasite which is inborn or inherited, and not acquired.

Naval Ill Syn 'Joint Ill' in foals.

Neck Its main function is to support the head, for which special provision is made by the strong and powerful ligaments from the spines of the withers to the posterior part of the occipital bone.

Necrobacillosis Spherophorus necrophorus infection.

Necrosis Death of cells in a living individual. Necropsy is mostly used in veterinary medicine. Autopsy is mostly used in human medicine. It is local death of tissue within the living individual.

Necrotic enteritis A condition of unweaned and older pigs, characterized by scouring. The lesions are in the caecum and ileum.

■ **Necropsy/autopsy/P.M. Exam** It is examination of an individual after death by systemic dissection.

■ **Negative balance** An animal is in negative balance when it is secreting and/excreting more nutrients than it is receiving in its feed.

■ **Negri** bodies Intracytoplasmic,estrnophilic round inclusion bodies found in the brains of dogs and animals died of rabies.

■ **Neisseria** Spherical, Gram —negative bacteria, some of which are associated with eye infections.

■ **Nematode** Round worm.

■ **Nematodirus** parasitic worms of sheep.

■ **Nembutal** A white crystalline powder, soluble in water, and used for its narcotic and anaesthetic effects. Used to produce anaesthesia in all the domestic animals.

■ **Neomycin** Refers to antibiotic isolated from *Streptomyces fradiae.*

■ **Neonate** The newborn animal.

■ **Neoplasm** (New thing formed) Growth of new cells that proliferates without control, serves no useful function and has no orderly arrangement.

■ **Nephritis** Inflammation of kidneys.

■ **Nephrosis** Degenerative changes in the renal tubules.

■ **Nephrectomy** is the name given to the operation by which one of the kidneys is removed.

■ **Nephrolithiasis** means the presence of a stone in the pelvis of the kidney.

■ **Nephrotomy** means the operation of cutting into the kidney.

■ **Nerve** Bundle of motor and or sensory nerve-fibres with accompanying connective tissue and blood vessels, in a common sheath of connective tissue.

■ **Nervous system** It is the system that receives the information with regard to the changes in the environment of the body, and in response regulates appropriate function.

■ **Net energy** This is that part of metabolisable energy over the use of which the animal has complete control.

■ **Net protein ratio** The difference between the average final body weight of a test group of animals fed a protein diet and that of control group receiving a protein free diet, divided by the amount of protein taken by the test group.

■ **Neuralgia** Sharp pain alongwith the course of a nerve.

■ **Neurectomy** is an operation in which part of a nerve is excised. The operation is sometimes performed to give relief from incurable lameness.

■ **Neuritis** Inflammation of nerve.

■ **Neuroglia** These are supporting interstitial cells of nervous tissue.

■ **Neuron** A nerve cell. The functional unit of nervous system.

■ **Neuronophagia** Engulfing of dead/necrotic tissue by glial cells.

■ **Neurology** That branch of medical science which deals with the nervous system.

■ **Neurotrauma** Mechanical injury to a nerve.

■ **Neurotoxin** A chemical that is poisonous to the nervous system.

■ **Neutral** Indifferent

■ **Neutralise** To remove the excess acidity from a dairy product usually cream or ice cream mix.

■ **Neutraliser** Alkaline substance for controlling milk acidity. Neutralisers permitted under PFA Rules are sodium hydroxide, sodium bicarbonate.

■ **Neutron** An uncharged particle in the nucleus of an atom.

■ **Neutropenia** decrease number of neutrophils in blood.

■ **Neutrophil** Also called polymorphonuclear leukocyte; a highly phagocytic granulocyte.

■ **Neutrophilia** An increase in the total number of neutrophils in the blood.

■ **Newcastle disease** Syn Ranikhet disease of poultry.

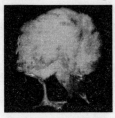

NEWCASTLE DISEASE

- **New forest disease** A painful eye condition which can lead to blindness if neglected.

- **Niacin** Nicotinic acid. Its deficiency causes pellagra, Vitamin of B group.

- **Nicking** The production of progeny that are superior to the parents which produce them. It is sometimes referred to as heterosis.

- **Nicotine** It is the main alkaloid which occurs in tobacco leaves.

- **Nicotinic acid** A component of vitamin B_2, present in yeast, meat, eggs, milk, etc. Deficiency causes Black Tongue.

- **Nictitating membrane** Third eyelid, transparent fold of skin, lies at inner (anterior) corner of eye or below lower eyelid.

- **Night blindness** Caused by Vitamin A deficiency (Nyctalopia).

- **Nisin** A polypeptide bacteriocin (antimicrobial substance) produced by *Streptococcus lactis*. Naturally present in small quantities in some milk.

- **NIT** Egg of louse or other parasitic insect.

- **Nitrites** are salts which, in excess, convert haemoglobin into methaemoglobin, may cause death from lack of oxygen.

- **Nitrofurazone** A drug of value in the control of coccidiosis.

- **Nitrofuran** A synthetic antimicrobial drug.

- **Nitrogen free extract** That part of feed dry matter which is not crude protein, crude fat, crude fibre, or ash. It consists mostly of sugars and starches. Sometimes referred to as NFE.

- **Nitrosamines** They are very powerful chemical carcinogens. They cause cancer of specific organs.

- **Node** means a localised swelling generally upon a bone or nerve fibre.

- **Nogalamycin** Antineoplastic antibiotic produced by *Streptomyces nogalater*.

- **Nomenclature** The system of naming things.

- **Nondisjunction** The failure of a pair of sister (homologous) chromosomes to separate in the reductional division of meiosis.

■ **Noninfectious** disease Which is caused by injury, vegetable or mineral poison, heat or cold, faulty nutrition, abnormal physiology, or abnormal tissue growth.

■ **Nonprotein** Any one of a group of ammoniacal nitrogen containing compounds which are not true proteins. Urea is a common example.

■ **Non-sterioidal** anti inflammatory drug A drug, which is not based on a steriod nucleus. This drug is used to control the inflammatory response.

■ **Norm** a fixed or ideal standard.

■ **Normal** Agreeing with the regular and established type.

■ **Normal** saline is a solution of sodium chloride in sterile distilled water, which is isotonic with is about 0-9 per cent for mammals.

■ **Normoblast** is a red blood corpuscle which still contains the remnant of a nucleus.

■ **Normocyte** An erythrocyte having a normal diameter.

■ **Nose / Nasal cavity** It is the first part of the respiratory passage.

■ **Nostril** Syn Nose.

■ **Notifiable disease** Disease outbreaks which have to be notified to the police or government department concerned.

■ **Nourish** To feed an animal with substances necessary to life and growth.

■ **Nuclear** Pertaining to a nucleus.

■ **Nucleus** A spherical body (found within a cell) which contains the chromosomes on which the genes are located.

■ **Nucleotide** A chemical compound composed of a nitrogen base, a sugar, and a phosphoric acid molecule.

■ **Nulberry** Heart Disease Dietetic microangiopathy of pigs.

■ **Nulliparous** Females which have never given birth to young.

■ **Nutrient** The chemical substances found in feed materials which are necessary for the maintenance, production and health of animals.

■ **Nutriment** Anything that promotes growth or development.

■ **Nutrition** Various chemical reactions and physiological processes, which transform food into body tissues and activities, are called nutrition.

■ **Nutritionist** A specialist in the problems of nutrition.

■ **Nutritious** Substances which promote growth and participate in repairing tissues of the body.

■ **Nutritive ratio** The ratio between the digestible protein, and digestible non-nitrogenous nutrients.

■ **Nutritive value** It is the nutritional status of a feed or the per cent availability of nutrients from a feed. Milk is generally acknowledged as most nearly perfect single foodstuff.

■ **Nutritional roup** Presence of cheesy material in the eyes and nasal sinuses in birds which occurs due to vitamin A deficiency.

■ **Nux** vomica is the seed of the *Strychnos nuxvomica*. It has intensely bitter medicinal properties are due to two alkaloids.

■ **Nymph** Immature stage of an insect with incomplete metamorphosis.

■ **Nymphomania** Development of follicular cysts which result in prolonged oestrogen secretion and continued signs of proestrus or oestrus.

■ **Nystagmus** An involuntary oscillation of eyeball usually lateral.

❑

■ **Oat groat** Oat grain from which hull has been removed.

■ **Oats** (*Avena sativa*) A cultivated fodder crop; a rabi season forage cereal which requires climatic conditions similar to that of wheat and barley.

■ **Ob** Against; in front of.

■ **Obesity** Fatness in animal.

■ **Obligate anaerobes** They cannot grow or even survive without molecular oxygen are obligate aerobes.

■ **Obstetrics** is the art of the delivery of the young, and the study of the abnormalities and diseases.

■ **Octa** eight.

■ **Ocul** (o) eye.

■ **Ocular** Pertaining to the eye.

■ **Oedema** Accumulation of watery fluid in one or more of the body cavities or beneath the skin.

■ **Oesophageal groove** A groove in the wall of the stomach in ruminants connecting the oesophagus directly with the reticulum thus bypassing the rumen.

■ **Oesophagitis** Inflammation of the oesophagus.

■ **Oesophagus** The tube that connects the Pharynx to the stomach.

■ **Oesteoporosis** An abnormal porousness of bone as the result of a calcium, phosphorus, and/or vitamin D deficiency.

■ **Oestradiol** are hormones secreted by the ovary.

■ **Oestrogen** A female sex hormone secreted in the graaffian follicle and inducing heat or oestrus in the female animal.

■ **Oestroscope** It is an instrument for detecting oestrus or heat in cows.

■ **Oestrus** (Heat) Period The period during which the female shows desire for the male during which time oestrogens form graaffian follicle.

■ **Off feed** A term often used in reference to the condition of loss of appetite in farm animals.

- **Ohm** A unit of electric resistance.

- **Ointments** These are semi-solid, viscous substances which are applied locally to the skin or mucous membranes.

- **Old** aged, primitive.

- **Oleic acid** The principal unsaturated fatty acid of butterfat present upto 20–40 per cent.

- **Olfactory** Pertaining to the sense of smell.

- **Oligomenorrhoea** Infrequent menstruation with markedly diminished menstrual flow, relative amenorrhoea.

- **Oliguria** Reduced excretion of urine

- **Omasum** Syn 'Many Plies' or third stomach in ruminants. Used for crushing large particles of food.

- **Omnivorous** Feeding upon both plants and animals.

- **Oncogen** Refers to a substance that produces cancer.

- **Oncology** Science which deals with study of tumors.

- **Oocyst** An encysted sporozoan zygote in which cell division occurs to form the next infectious stage.

- **Oogenesis** The process by which egg cells are formed in the ovary of the female (gametogenesis in the females).

- **Oophorectomy** Syn 'Ovariectomy' or 'Spaying'. Removal of healthy ovary.

- **Oophoritis** Inflammation of ovary.

- **Operculum** Small piece of horny skin covering nostrils

- **Operation** any action performed with instruments or by the hands of a surgeon; a surgical procedure.

- **Ophthalmoscopy** Examination of the eye by means of the ophthalmoscope.

- **Opium** is the dried milky juice of the unripe seed-capsules of the White Indian Poppy—*Papaver somniferum.*

- **Opthalmoscope** an instrument containing a perforated mirror and lenses to examine the interior of the eye.

- **Opto** Visible; vision.

- **Ophthalmic** instillation Drugs inserted into the conjunctival sac.

- **Opthalmic** Pertaining to the eye.

- **Optic** Pertaining to the sense of sight.
- **Oral** By mouth
- **Oral contraceptives** Refer to the contraceptive agents that have been active after oral administration.
- **Orbit** The bony cavity which accommodates the eye ball is known as orbit.
- **Orchitis** Inflammation of testes.
- **Organ** An independent body part that performs a special function.
- **Organelle** Living substance in all the cells including mitochondria.
- **Organism** An individual living being plant or animal.
- **Organoleptic** properties Properties perceptible to the senses, especially taste and smell.
- **Origin** The source or beginning of anything.
- **Orth(o)** straight, normal, correct
- **Orgasm** The apex and culmination of sexual excitement.
- **Orifice** Entrance or outlet of any body cavity.
- **Ornithology** Study of birds.
- **Ornithosis** A virus disease of birds caused by the *Psittococis* group of organism.
- **OS** Top of the projected part of cervix through which cervical canal communicates with vagina.
- **Osleogenesis** Formation of bone.
- **Osmatic pressure** The force with which a solvent moves from a solution of lower solute concentration to a solution of higher solute concentration.
- **Osmosis** The diffusion through a semipermeable membrane, separating two liquid solutions. It tends to equalize their concentrations across the membrane.
- **Ossification** The process of bone formation is known as ossification.
- **Oste (o)** Bone
- **Osteoarthritis** Degenerative arthritis.
- **Osteoblast** A bone forming cell.
- **Osteoclast** Bone destroyer, the cell which dissolves or removes unwanted bone.

■ **Osteodystrophy** Diseases of bones in which there is failure of normal bone development, abnormal growth of bone which is already mature.

■ **Osteology** Scientific study of the bones.

■ **Osteotomy** Incision or transaction of a bone.

■ **Ostertagiasis** Infestation with species of Ostertagia worms, which produce gastroentritis.

■ **Osteomalacia** Removal of Ca salts from the already formed bones.

■ **Osteomyelitis** Inflammation of the bone marrow.

■ **Osteophagia** Chewing of bones by the animals.

■ **Osteoporosis** Loss of bone density caused by excessive absorption of calcium and phosphorus from the bone.

■ **OTC** Over the counter, the drugs not required by law to be sold on prescription only.

■ **Otology** Branch of medicine dealing with the ear.

■ **Otorrhoea** Discharge of pus from the ears.

■ **Otoscope** An instrument for inspecting.

■ **Outcrossing** Mating unrelated animals generally within the same pure breed.

■ **Ovarian cyst** The ovary will form a fluid filled cyst on the surface of the ovary each month after an egg is released from the ovary during normal ovulation.

■ **Ovarian follicle** In mammals, the group of cells around the primary oocyte proliferate and form a surrounding noncellular layer.

■ **Ovarian wedge resection** The surgical removal of a portion of a polycystic ovary to induce ovulation.

■ **Ovario-ysterectomy** Removal of ovaries and uterus surgically.

■ **Ovary** The paired organs located just under the loin region of the female which produce the ova and release them into the infundibulum.

■ **Overdominance** The interaction of members of pair of genes (alleles) to produce a phenotypic effect that is superior in the heterozygote to either homozygote.

■ **Ovi** Ova, egg, ovum.

■ **Oviducts** (fallopian tube) Two tubes in the female

through which ovum (egg) moves from ovary to the cavity of uterus.

■ **Oviparous** Producing eggs that hatch after they have passed from the body of the parent.

■ **Ovular** Pertaining to an ovule or an ovum.

■ **Ovulation** It is the release of ovum from a mature graaffian follicle.

■ **Ovum** The mature reproductive cell or germ cell or gamete of the female which is produced in the ovaries.

■ **Ox** The domestic cattle, especially an adult castrated male used as a draught animal; bullock. (from Sanskrit Ushan).

■ **Oxacillin** Semi synthetic penicillin used as the sodium salt.

■ **Oxalate** Any salt of oxalic acid.

■ **Oxaluria** Excretion of urine, containing calcium oxalate crystals, associated often **with dyspepsia.**

■ **Oxidation** Chemically, the increase of positive charges on an atom or the loss of negative charges.

■ **Oxidized flavour** Defect in milk due to fat oxidation.

■ **Oxyclozanide** A drug for use to sheep and cattle against liver-flukes.

■ **Oxytetracycline** An antibiotic.

■ **Oxyphenbutazone** Non steroid anti-inflammatory agent.

■ **Oxytocin** A hormone secreted by the posterior pituitary gland and also by the corpus luteum which brings 'milk let down' mechanism and also stimulates contraction of muscles of the uterus.

■ **Oxyuris** is another name for the thread worm.

■ **Oyster shell flour** Oyster shell is a hard shell of a shell fish found especially on the bottom of the sea.

❏

P/P

- **P.U.O.** Pyrexia of unknown origin.
- **PABA** Para-aminobenzoic acid; a precursor for folic acid synthesis.
- **Pail feeding** Milk feeding to calves in buckets.
- **Palatability** Acceptability of a feed, influencing the amount eaten.
- **Palate** Roof of vertebrate mouth.
- **Palatitis** (Lampas) Inflammation of palate.
- **Pale (o)** old, yellow.
- **Palmar** The surface of the fore limb that contacts the ground
- **Palomino** A golden coat color in horses with the mane and tail a light-blond or silvery color.
- **Palpation** Feeling the surface with hand to determine the condition of a normal or diseased organ.
- **Pancreas** A large, elongated gland located near the stomach. It is partly an endocrine gland producing hormone (Insulin) and partly an

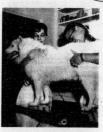

PALPATION

exocrine gland producing the pancreatic juice for digestion of food in the intestines.

- **Pancreatic juice** Digestive juice which gets produced by the pancreas and secreted into the duodenum.
- **Pantothenic acid** Vitamin of B group, forming a coenzyme. Occurs in rice bran and plant and animal tissues.
- **Papilla** A small nipple-like or pimple-like projection.
- **Papillomatosis** The common wart of cattle and horses, is transmissible by intradermal injection and is caused by a virus with considerable host specificity.
- **Papule** Circumscribed elevation of the skin.

- **Para grass** A grass that is native of South America and West Africa; grown as fodder grass in various parts of India.

- **Parakeratosis** Parakeratosis is a conditon of the skin in which keratinization of the epithelial cells is incomplete.

- **Paralumbar** Injection Injection of a solution of a local anesthetic about the lumbar nerves as they leave the spinal column.

- **Paralysis** Complete immobility of muscles.

- **Parametritis** Inflammation of suspensary ligaments of uterus only.

- **Paraphimosis** Condition in which extended penis cannot be retracted back due to inflammatory swelling.

- **Parasite** A disease-causing organism that lives in an organic relationship within or upon another living organism.

- **Parasympathetic** (nervous system) A subdivison of the autonomic nervous system whose centres are located in the brain and lower portion of the spinal cord. Its action is inhibitory.

- **Parasympatholytic drug** Refers to a drug that is able to block the actions of the parasympathetic nervous system and of parasympathomimetic drugs.

- **Parathyroid glands** These are four reddish yellow coloured small bodies situated at variable positions, close to the thyroid gland.

- **Parental generation** The first generation of a genetic experiment. Individuals in the first generation are often considered to be pure or homozygous.

- **Parenteral** administration Literally this term is used for administration other than by the gut. However, it has been usually taken to mean administration by injection.

- **Paresis** Incomplete immobility of muscles.

- **Parotitis** Inflammation of any of the salivary glands.

- **Parrot mouth** A malformation of the mouth in which the lower jaw is shorter than the upper jaw.

- **Parthenogenus** When development of ovum starts without entry of sperm, it may be due to temporary shock, electoral stimuli etc.

■ **Partial dominance** A situation where a gene is not completely, but partially, dominant to its own allele.

■ **Parturition** It is the process of giving birth to young ones.

■ **Passive immunity** Refers to the temporary but immediate specific immunity which is acquired by injection of the appropriate antibody or of serum containing it.

■ **Pasteurization** A heat treatment process which secures destruction of pathogenic organisms without impairing the commercial value of milk.

■ **Patchymeningitis** Inflammation of durameter.

■ **Patella** This is a triangular sesamoid bone placed in front of the trochlea of femur.

■ **Pathogen** A microorganism that produces a disease.

■ **Pathogenesis** Progression of disease process from its initiation to its termination whether in recovery or death.

■ **Pathogenicity** The capacity to produce disease.

■ **Pathology** Study of the anatomical, chemical or physiological alterations in an organism as a result of disease.

■ **Pad (ped)** A cushion-like mass of soft material.

■ **Pain** a feeling of distress, suffering, or agony, caused by stimulation of specialized nerve endings.

■ **Pam** Pyridine –2-aldoxime methiodide. This has been recommended as an antidote to be given intravenously.

■ **Pant (o)** All, the whole.

■ **Paraffin** is the general term used to designate a series of saturated hydrocarbons.

■ **Parameter** Variable whose measure is indicative of a quantity or function that cannot itself be precisely determined by direct methods.

■ **Paraplegia** means paralysis of the posterior pair of limbs, may be accompanied paralysis of the muscles which control the passage of urine and faeces to the outside.

■ **Parasitism** The association of two organisims, one of which benefits by nourishing itself at the expense of the other.

■ **Parathion** Agricultural insecticide toxic to humans and animals.

■ **Parotid** Near the ear.

■ **Particle** A tiny mass of material.

■ **Paste** A semisolid Preparation, generally.

■ **Pasteurella** is the name for organisms of the haemorrhagic septicaemia group, the diseases they produce are called 'pasteurellosis'.

PASTEURELLA MULTOCIDA

■ **Pathogenic** Disease producing.

■ **Pathy** Morbid condition or disease.

■ **Patient** A person who is ill or is undergoing treatment for disease.

■ **Pause** An interruption, or rest.

■ **Peat** scours a name given in Australia and Canada to molybdenum poisoning in grazing cattle.

■ **Peck order** This is the equivalent in poultry of the order of precedence.

■ **Pectoral** Pertaining to the chest.

■ **Pectoral** Region of body bearing forelimbs.

■ **Pedigree** The record of an individual's ancestry.

■ **Ped (o)** Foot.

■ **Pediatrics** That branch of medicine dealing with child and its development, diseases of child and their treatment.

■ **Pediculosis** Infestation of body with lice.

■ **Pellets** Compacted particles of feed formed by forcing ground material through die openings.

■ **Pelvic** Region of body bearing hind-limbs.

■ **Penetrance** The percentage of times a gene is expected to be expressed in the phenotype that it is expressed.

■ **Penicillins** A group of antibiotics produced either by Penicillium (natural penicillins) or by adding side chains to the β–lactam ring (semisynthetic penicillins).

■ **Pellegra** Rough skin caused by Niacin deficiency (Vit. B)

■ **Pelvis** The lower portion of the trunk of the body.

■ **Penicillinase** A penicillin destroying enzyme produced by certain bacteria, e.g. *E. coli*.

■ **Penis** This is a cylindrical structure and the organ of copulation.

■ **Pentobarbital sodium** A narcotic and anaesthetic. (see Nembutal).

■ **Peptide** A chain of two (di-), three (tri-), or more (poly-) amino acids.

■ **Peptone** Short chains of amino acids produced by the action of acids or enzymes on proteins.

■ **Per** Throughout, completely, extremely.

■ **Perch** Means raised iron or wooden bars provided for poultry to sit on.

■ **Percussion** The body surface is struck so as to set deep parts in vibration and cause them to emit audible sounds.

■ **Pericarditis** Inflammation of the pericardium.

■ **Pericardium** It is the covering of heart.

■ **Perimetritis** Inflammation of serosal layer of uterus only.

■ **Perineum** the region lying between the anus and the genital organs in the male, between the anus and the mammary region in the female.

■ **Period** An interval or division of time.

■ **Periodic** Recurring at regular intervals of time.

■ **Periople** It is a soft, flat, light coloured band which surrounds the coronary border of the hoof.

■ **Periosteum** Bones are covered by a membrane called periosteum.

■ **Periphery** An outward surface.

■ **Perirectal** Around the rectum.

■ **Peristalsis** The wormlike movement by which the alimentary canal contracts.

■ **Peristaltic movement** Contraction of smooth muscles like intestines.

■ **Peritoneal cavity** Abdominal cavity.

■ **Peritoneum** It is a serous membrane which lines the abdominal walls.

■ **Peritonitis** Inflammation of the peritoneum or membrane lining the abdominal and pelvic cavities and covering the contained viscera.

■ **Permanent teeth** Eruptions of permanent teeth starts from the age of one year and become completed by 3 to 4 years.

■ **Permeability** The extent to which substances dissolved in the body fluids are able to pass through the membranes of cells or layers of cell e.g. walls of capillary blood vessels or secretory or absorptive tissues.

■ **Pernicious anaemia** R.B.C. fail to proliferate and mature.

■ **Peroxidase** A heat-resistant enzyme catalysing the oxidation of substances in the presenece of hydrogen peroxide.

■ **Peroxide** That oxide of any element containing more oxygen than any other.

■ **Pessary** Refers to a dosage from, a medicated suppository, for insertion into the vagina.

■ **Petechia** small spots on the surface of an organ or the skin, generally red or purple in colour.

■ **Pethidine** An analgesic (pain relieves) used for dogs and cats.

■ **Petri dish** A shallow circular glass dish with lid in which bacteria are grown on a solid medium.

■ **pH** A symbol used to express acidity or alkalinity.

■ **Phagocytes** Cells in the body (leucocytes) which ingest and destroy foreign particles or other infectious agents in the body.

■ **Phagocytosis** It is the process by which foreign particles, including bacteria, are ingested by leucocytes and by certain endothelial cells of the body.

■ **Phalaris** staggers Poisoning due to ingestion of *phalaris spp.*

■ **Pharmacognosy** It is concerned with the sources and the physical and chemical properties of drugs of vegetable and animal origin.

■ **Pharmaco-kinetics** The study of the way in which drugs are absorbed, distributed and excreted from the body.

■ **Pharmacology** Refers to the branch of medical science

that deals with the mechanisms of action, use and unwanted effects of drugs.

■ **Pharmacopoeia** An authoritative treatise on drugs and their preparations.

■ **Pharmacy** It is an additional field which is included in pharmacology with the collection, preparation, standardization, and dispensing of drugs.

■ **Pharyngitis** Pharyngitis is inflammation of the pharynx.

■ **Pharynx** It is roughly a funnel shaped space at the base of the cranial cavity and behind the posterior nasal apertures.

■ **Phenocopy** The production of a particular phenotype by environment that is also produced by heredity.

■ **Phenol Coefficient** The ratio of the killing power of the disinfectant to the killing power of pure phenol when determined under standard conditions.

■ **Phenomenon** Any sign or objective symptom or any observable occurance or fact.

■ **Phenothiazine** A pale greenish grey powder which darkens on exposure to light. Phenothiazine is an anthelmintic.

■ **Phenotype** The observable, visible or measurable characteristics of an individual without reference to its genetic constitution.

■ **Phenylbutazone** An analgesic for the relief of pain, associated with inflammation of joints and muscles.

■ **Phimosis** Condition in which penis cannot be extended from the prepuce due to inflammation.

■ **Phlebitis** Inflammation of vein

■ **Phlebotmus** A genus of biting sand flies, the females of which suck blood.

■ **Phlebotomy** is the name for the operation of cutting a vein so that blood my be drawn.

■ **Phlegmon/cellulitis** Diffuse suppurative inflammation in which infection spreads further to dermis and subcutaneous tissue.

■ **Phosphatase test** A test to determine heat treatment efficiency in the pasteurization of milk.

■ **Phospholipids** Lipids containing phosphoric acid and nitrogenous bases, important factor in auto-oxidation of milk fat and development of oiliness and cardboard flavour. Lecithin, cephalin and sphingomyelin are the phospholipids in milk.

■ **Phot(o)** Light.

■ **Photochemistry** The study of plant chemistry.

■ **Photogenic** Produced by light.

■ **Photophobia** means a codition in which animal, suffering from inflammation in the eye objects to a strong light falling upon. Fear of light.

■ **Photosensetization** Dermatitis produced by the action of sunlight on certain photodynamic substances present in the skin.

■ **Photosensitivity** The term used for the abnormal reactivity of the skin to sunlight, giving rise to erythema, rash, blisters, etc.

■ **Phycology** The study of algae.

■ **Phylum** A taxonomic classification between kingdom and class.

■ **Physical** Pertaining to the body, to material things.

■ **Physician** An authorized practitioner of medicine.

■ **Physicochemical** Pertaining to both physics and chemistry.

■ **Physics** Study of the laws and phenomena of nature. Especially of forces and general properties of matter and energy.

■ **Physio** Nature.

■ **Physiology** Study of the processes occuring in living organism.

■ **Phyt(o)** Plant.

■ **Phytogenous** Derived from plants.

■ **Piamater** This is a more delicate membrane, closely invests the brain and spinal cord.

■ **Pica** Means depraved appetite and chewing of materials other than normal food i.e. bones, sticks, stones etc.

■ **Piebald** A black and white spotted horse.

■ **Pigment** Any colouring matter of body

■ **Pili, Pill** A small globular or oval medicated mass to be swallowed.

- **Piliconcretion** or hair balls Concretions of hairs in the stomach.

- **Pills** Result from mixing powdered drugs with sticky substances such as honey or glucose, molding a given weight of this sticky mass and coating it with an inert ingredient.

- **Pilocarpine** The chief use is in the treatment of impaction or stoppage of the intestines. A cholinergic alkaloid.

- **Pimply Gut** Presence of nectrotic nodules in the wall of intestines due to *oesophagostomum spp.*

- **Pineal gland** It is a cone shaped grey body situated in a deep recess of mid-brain.

- **Pink-eye** is the colloquial name for infectious keratitis of cattle caused by *Moraxella.*

- **Pinto** A horse with dark spots (any colour) on a white background.

- **Pinworm** Any oxyurid.

- **Piperazine** compounds are used in the treatment of roundworm infestations.

- **Piroplasms** are protozoon parasites of the red-blood corpuscles and the cause of numerous tick-transmitted diseases.

- **Pisces** Fishes.

- **Pituitary gland** A gland at the base of the brain (also called master gland of the body).

- **Pituitrin** Trademark for a preparation of posterior pituitary injection.

- **Pityriasis** Pityriasis or dandruff is a condition characterized by the presence of bran-like scales on the skin surface.

- **Placebo** An inactive substance or preparation given to satisfy the patient's symbolic need for drug therapy.

- **Placenta** Covering of the foetus in the uterine horn.

- **Placentophagy** Ingetion of fetal membrane. It is common in bitches.

- **Planter** The contact surface of the hind limb in standing condition

- **Plasma** Plasma is the liquid remaining after extraction of the cellular elements of blood.

- **Plasma membrane** The selectively permeable membrane enclosing the cytoplasm of a cell; the outer layer in animal cells, internal to the cell wall in other organisms.

■ **Plasmodium** A multinucleated mass of protoplasm, as in plasmodial slime molds or When written as a genus, refers to the protozoan agent of malaria.

■ **Plastic** capable of being molded, a substance produced by chemical condensation or by polymerization.

■ **Plate** A flat structure or layer, as a thin layer of bone.

■ **Platform test** A rapid test made at the milk receiving platform of a dairy to determine milk quality.

■ **Platinum** A Chemical element.

■ **Pledge** A solemn statement of intention.

■ **Pleitrophy** A situation where one gene affects two or more traits.

■ **Pleo** More.

■ **Pleoriperaus** Animal which has calved more than one.

■ **Pleura** Serous membrane covering the lung and lining the inner wall of the thorax.

■ **Pleurisy** Inflammation of the pleura.

■ **Pleurotomy** Incision of the pleura.

■ **Plexus** A network of interlaced nerves or blood vessels.

■ **Plug** An obstructing mass.

■ **Plutonium** A Chemical element.

■ **Pneo** breath, breathing.

■ **Pneumograph** An instrument for recording respiratory movements.

■ **Pneumonia** Inflammation of lungs

■ **Pneumonitis** Interstitial pneumonia

■ **Pneumothorax** Entry of air into the pleural cavity in sufficient quantity.

■ **Pock** A pustule, especially of smallpox.

■ **Pod** (o) Foot.

■ **Poikolocytosis** Variation in shape of R.B.C.

■ **Point** A small area or spot, the sharp end of an object.

■ **Poison** A substance, which on ingestion, inhalation, absorption, application, injection, or development within the body, in relatively small amount, may cause structural damage or functional disturbance.

■ **Poliomalacia** Softening of grey matter.

■ **Poll** Region between the ears or a little behind them.

■ **Polled** Cattle without horn by birth.

■ **Poly** Many, much.

■ **Polyandry** Mating of one female with many males.

■ **Polycythaemia** Increase in number of circulating R.B.C.

■ **Polydipsia** Excessive water intake

■ **Polyestrous cycle** Reproductive cycle which occurs several times a year.

■ **Polygalactia** Excessive secretion of milk.

■ **Polygenic inheritance** A trait which is determined by many pairs of genes. It is also referred to as multiple gene inheritance.

■ **Polymer** A molecule consisting of a sequence of similar units or monomers.

■ **Polymyositis** Inflammation of groups of muscles which manifests as muscle weakness.

■ **Polyneuritis** Inflammation of nerves or their sheaths occuring in different parts of the body at the same time.

■ **Polyploidy** The duplication of chromosomes in body cells so that the individual possesses 3n or 4n, etc. numbers of chromosomes.

■ **Polyspermy** Entry of more than one sperm into the ovum.

■ **Polyuria** Increased excretion of urine.

■ **Polyvalent vaccine** One prepared from cultures of several strains of the same bacterial or viral. Single vaccine can now protect agaisnt eight diseases.

■ **Pons** It is a transverse prominence situated in front and ventral to medulla oblongata.

■ **Popping** Action of the rapid application of dry heat, causing a sudden expansion of the grain which ruptures the endosperm.

■ **Posology** It is a study of dosage of medicine.

■ **Post** is a prefix signifying after or behind.

■ **Posterior** directed toward or situated at the back, opposite of anterior.

■ **Postmenopausal** Occurring after the menopause.

■ **Postoperative** After a surgical operation.

■ **Post-partum** Following the birth of a young one.

■ **Postpartum anoestrus** Not coming to heat after parturition.

■ **Posture** an attitude of the body.

■ **Potable** Fit to drink.

■ **Potash**, or Potassa is the popular name for carbonate of potassium.

■ **Potassium** is a metal which, on account of its great affinity for other substances. Potassium is a mineral element essential for the body. Its content in body fluids is controlled by the kidneys.

■ **Potency Power**, <gynaecology> The ability of the male to perform sexual intercourse. <pharmacology> The power of a medicinal agent to produce the desired effects. <anatomy> The ability of an embryonic part to develop and complete its destiny.

■ **Potentiate** To make more potent.

■ **Potentiation** Enhancement of the agent by another so that the combined effect is greater than the sum of the effects of each one alone.

■ **Potentiative** It is the tissue response to simultaneously given drugs that produce an effect greater than the sum of their separate actions.

■ **Pouch** Pocket like space or sac.

■ **Poultice** The poultice is a soft, pasty preparation for application to the surface of the body, with the purpose of irritation.

■ **Power** Capability, potency.

■ **Pox** a group of diseases caused by members of the Poxvirus group.

■ **PPLO** Pleuropneumonia like organisms.

■ **PPM** Parts per million.

■ **PPR** 'Peste des petitis ruminants' is a disease of goats and sheep.

■ **Practice** The utilization of one's knowledge in a particular profession.

■ **Pre molars** Teeth followed by canine teeth.

■ **Precipitate** To cause settling in solid particles of substance in solution.

■ **Precursor** A compound that can be used by the body to form another compound. Something that precedes. In biological processes, a substance form which another, usually more active or mature substance is formed.

■ **Predator** An animal that preys upon other animals for its food.

■ **Predisposing** causes Those causes which make the animal susceptible to the disease.

■ **Predisposition** A latent susceptibility to disease which may be activated under certain conditions.

■ **Prednisolone** Drug which raises blood-sugar levels and has been used in the treatment of agalactia.

■ **Pregnancy** toxaemia of sheep See ketosis.

■ **Prehension** The seizing (grasping) and conveying of food to the mouth.

■ **Premature birth** Birth of a youngone before full term.

■ **Premenstrual** Occurring before menstruation.

■ **Premix** A uniform mixture of one or more nutrients and additives diluent and / or carried.

■ **Premolars** Crushing teeth of mammals, having usually more than one root and a pattern of ridges and *projections of* bitting surface.

■ **Premunition** A type of resistance that develops due to the presence of a residual infection of a protozoan parasite in the body.

■ **Prepotent** The ability of a parent to stamp its characteristics on its offspring so that they resemble that parent, or each other more than usual.

■ **Prepuce** The foreskin or skin covering the end of the penis.

■ **Prescription** A prescription is an order to a pharmacist written by a veterinarian, physician, or dentist to prepare the prescribed medicine, to affix the directions.

■ **Presentation** means the appearance in parturition of some particular part of the young animal's body at the cervix of the womb.

■ **Preservative** Any material that prevents decomposition, fermentation, spoilage and decay.

■ **Prestratification method** A process of ghee making from desi butter by heating.

■ **Prevalence** This is defined as the number of cases of disease or infection existing at any given time in relation to the unit of population in which they occur.

■ **Primaquine** A compound used as an antimalarial.

■ **Primary dysmenorrhoea** Painful menses due to a functional disturbance and not due to organic factors such as growths, inflammation or anatomy.

■ **Primary oocyte** The enlarging ovum before maturity is reached, as opposed to the secondary oocyte or polar body.

■ **Primiparous** Which is calving first time.

■ **Primitive** First in point of time.

■ **Probang** A rod of flexible material designed to aid removal of foreign bodies from the oesophagus.

■ **Probiotics** Preparations containing live micro-organisms.

■ **Product** The substance formed in a chemical reaction.

■ **Production disease** Metabolic diseases attributable to the imbalance between rate of input of dietary nutrients and output of production.

■ **Profile** a simple outline as a graph representing quantitatively a set of characteristics.

■ **Proflavine** A constituent of acriflavine.

■ **Progeny** Offspring .

■ **Progestagens** These drugs are used to control breeding and have a progesterone like action.

■ **Progesterone** A hormone produced by the corpus luteum and by the placenta which inhibits the action of estrogen and assist in developing the mammary system.

■ **Prognosis** Is a forecast of the probable outcome of an attack of disease.

■ **Prolactin** A hormone associated with lactation and secreted by the pituitary gland.

■ **Prolapse** means the slipping down of some organ or structure. The term is applied to the displacements of the rectum and female generative organs.

■ **Promazine** a phenothiazine derivative used as a major tranquilizer.

■ **Promazine** hydrochloride An effective sedative and pre-narcotic.

■ **Promethazine** A phenothiazine derivative, hydrochloride salt is used as an antihistaminic.

■ **Prophase** The first stage of mitosis in which the chromosomes become shortened and thickened in appearance, the nuclear membrane disappears, and the spindle fibers become polarized.

■ **Prophylaxis** Means any "treatment" that is adopted with a view to the warding-off of disease.

■ **Proprietary** Denoting a medicine protected against free competition as to name, composition, or manufacturing process by patent, trademark, copyright, or secrecy.

■ **Prostaglandins** A large group of chemically related 20-carbon hydroxy fatty acids with variable physiological effects in the body.

■ **Prostate gland** A gland in male mammals surrounding the urethra, near the bladder.

■ **Protectives** and adsorbents Insoluble, inert and finely ground substances applied to prevent friction and absorb toxins and exudative wastes.

■ **Protein** A chemical molecule composed of chains of amino acids.

■ **Proteinuria** Presence of protein in the urine.

■ **Proteolysis** It is a process of breaking down of complex proteins by protease enzymes.

■ **Proteolytic** An enzyme capable of hydrolyzing a protein.

■ **Proteus** A genus of bacteria. Proteus species are common pathogens affecting the urinary system.

■ **Proteus** Genus of gram-negative, motile bacteria.

■ **Prothrombin** A substance formed in the liver with the assistance of vitamin K, and essential for the clotting of blood.

■ **Proton** A positively charged particle in the nucleus of an atom.

■ **Protozoa** Unicellular organism belonging to the kingdom protista.

TRICHOMONAS

- **Proven sire** One having adequate number of measured progeny.

- **Proventriculus** Anterior part of stomach of birds where enzymes are secreted.

- **Proximal** Upper or superior.

- **Pruritus** Intense itching.

- **Pseud(o)** false.

- **Pseudocowpox** Mild infection of udder and teats caused by virus.

- **Pseudo pregnancy** In it, the physical signs of pregnancy are exhibited in the absence of foetus or foetuses.

- **Psittocosis** A disease of parrots and man caused by a virus.

- **Psoriasis** A chronic skin disease characterized by scaly patches.

- **Psyche** the mind; human faculty for thought, judgment and emotion.

- **Psychiatry** That branch of medicine dealing with the study, treatment, and prevention of mental illness.

- **Psychology** The science dealing with mind and mental processes, especially in relation to human and animal behaviour.

- **Ptyalin**–See Amylase.

- **Puberty** The age at which the reproductive organs of the animal becomes functional.

- **Pubis** A pair of bones forming the floor of the birth canal.

- **Pullet** A young hen less than a year old.

- **Pullorum disease of chicks** (Bacillary white diarrhoea) Acute, infectious, and fatal disease of chicks caused by *Salmonella pullorun*.

- **Pulmonary** Pertaining to the lungs.

- **Pulmonary** circulation Blood supply to lungs.

- **Pulp** Soft, juicy animal or vegetable tissue.

- **Pulpy kidney** Acute toxaemia of ruminants caused by proliferation of Clostridium perfringens type D in intestine & liberation of toxins.

- **Pulse** (Zool) A rhythmical dilation of the artery cuased by the systolic output of the heart.

- **Pump** An apparatus for drawing or forcing liquids or gases.

- **Puncture** the act of piercing or penetrating with a pointed object, or instrument; a wound so made.

- **Pupa** Stage usually dormant, between the larva and the adult of insects having complete metamorphosis.

- **Pupil** The central aperture of the iris through which light passes to, reach retina of eyes.

- **Pure bred** An animal whose ancestry can be traced back through all lines of the foundation animals of the breed.

- **Pure culture** A population of one strain or species of bacteria.

- **Purgatives** are which gently stimulate the bowels and render the evacuation more frequent.

- **Purified** diet A mixture of the known essential dietary nutrient in a pure form that is fed to experimental (test) animals in nutrition studies.

- **Purines** The class of nucleic acid bases that includes adenine and guanine.

- **Purpura** Haemorrhagica This is an acute, non-contagious disease, occurring chiefly in the horse, and characterized by extensive, oedematous and haemorrhagic swellings of subcutaneous tissues, accompanied by haemorrhages in the mucosae and viscera.

- **Purulent** Pertaining to pus.

- **Pus** This thick, often yellowish fluid, found abscesses and sinuses, and on the surfaces of ulcers and inflamed areas where the skin is broken.

- **Pustule** Focal area of suppurative inflammation of skin confined to epidermis.

- **Putrefaction** The decomposition of proteins by microorganisms under anaerobic conditions.

- **Putrid** butter A flavour defect in butter, result of protein decomposition of certain species of putrefactive bacteria. Butter made from sweet, unripened cream and light salt butter are very susceptible to putrid flavour.

- **PVP-I** Povidone-iodine.

- **Pyaemia** Presence of pus in blood stream.

- **Pyelonephritis** Clinically it is characterized by pyuria, suppurative nephritis, cystitis and ureteritis.

■ **Pyknosis** Shrinking and condensation of nuclear material.

■ **Pyo**–is a prefix attached to the names diseases to indicate the presence of pus.

■ **Pyo** pus.

■ **Pyoderma** Pustular condition of the skin.

■ **Pyogenic** Term applied to those bacteria which causes the formation of pus and so lead to the production of abscesses.

■ **Pyometra** Accumulation of pus in uterus.

■ **Pyorrhoea** Purulent inflammation of the gum.

■ **Pyosalpinx** Accumulation of pus in the fallopian tube.

■ **Pyretic** Pertaining to fever.

■ **Pyrexia** means fever.

■ **Pyridoxine** Vitamins B$_6$.

■ **Pyrimidines** The class of nucleic acid bases that includes uracil, thymine, and cytosine.

■ **Pyro** Fire; heat.

■ **Pyrogens** Substances which are produced by living bacteria. They cause a rise inbody temperature on injection.

■ **Pyuria** Presence of pus in the urine

❑

- **Q. Fever** Caused by *Coxiella brunetii* in cattle and man causing patchy nodular lesions in visceral organs.

- **q.3.h** every three hours

- **q.d.** *qua'que di'e* (every day)

- **q.h.** *qua'que ho'ra* (every hour)

- **q.i.d.** *qua'ter in di'e* (four times a day).

- **q.s.** *quan'tum so'tis* as much as needed (a sufficient amount)

- **qt** quart.

- **Quack** one who misrepresents his ability and experience in diagnosis and treatment of disease.

- **Quadriceps** means having four heads.

- **Quadriplegia** Paralysis of all four limbs.

- **Qualitative traits** Traits determined by many genes which have no sharp distinction among phenotypes. Environmental factors often greatly affect such traits.

- **Quarantine** Implies governmental regulations for the prevention of the spread of infectious disease by which an animal or animals which have come from infected countries or areas are detained at the frontiers or ports of entrance or at other official centres for a period of isolation before being allowed to mix with the stock of the country.

- **Quarg** Fresh cheese, associated with Germany. Known as Tvorog in Eastern Europe. Represents a wide range of sour milk curd products.

- **Quaternary ammonium compounds** (QACs) Non-corrosive and odourless disinfectants, with an advantage over hypoclorites.

- **Quinine** An antimalarial drug derived from the cinchona tree and effective against schizogony stage of parasite in red blood cells.

- **Quinolines** Drugs having a quinoline nucleus in their molecules.

- **Quotient** A number obtained by division.

Rabies Viral disease (Latin word for Madness) Is a specific inoculable contagious disease of virtually all mammals including man and occasionally it occurs in birds.

Racketic rosary Enlarged costo condral junctions due to rickets.

Radical Directed to the root or cause.

Radicle One of the smallest branches of a vessel or nerve.

Radioactive Giving off atomic energy in the form of alpha, beta, or gamma rays.

Radiobiology Science dealing with the effect of radiation on living organisms.

Radioisotope A radioactive form of an element.

Radiology the branch of medical science dealing with use of radiant energy in diagnosis and treatment of disease.

Radium Radioactive element.

Radius It is larger but not longer bone. It is situated in a vertical direction, forms elbow joint with the humerus above and carpal joint with the carpal bones below.

Rage State of violent anger.

Rale An abnormal respiratory sound heard on auscultation, indicating some pathologic condition.

Ram Male sheep.

Ramification Distribution in branches.

Rancid A term used to describe fats that have undergone partial decomposition.

Rancidity A flavour defect in milk due to oxidation and hydrolysis of fat by lipases.

Random mating A system of mating where each male has the equal opportunity of mating with any female in the group.

Ranikhet disease Also known as Newcastle Disease. It is Infectious, contagious and highly fatal disease caused by a virus. Affects birds of all ages.

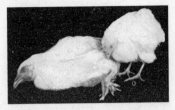

RANIKHET DISEASE

- **Ranula** Dilatation of salivary gland at the floor of the mouth containing clear fluid.

- **Rate** The speed or frequency with which an event or circumstance occurs per unit of time.

- **Ratio** An expression of the quantity of one substance entity in relation to that of another.

- **Ration** It is a twenty-four hr. allowance of a feed or mixture of feeding stuffs.

- **Ration balanced** A balanced ration is one which will supply the various nutrients in such proportions as will properly nourish a given animal when fed in proper amounts for a 24 hours period.

- **Ration, maintenance** The amount of feed required to maintain an animal when at rest and not yielding milk or work.

- **Rational** Based upon reason.

- **React** To respond to a stimulus

- **Reaction** The response to stimuli.

- **Reading** Understanding of written or printed symbols representing words.

- **Reagent** Substance used to produce a chemical reaction so as to detect, measure, produce etc.

- **Reaing** Respiratory noise produced due to paralysis of vocal cords.

- **Rearing** To look after, to shelter or bring up.

- **Reception** A comprehensive term for the whole process of receiving, checking, testing, recording, tipping and pumping away of raw milk at a depot.

- **Recessive gene** A gene whose phenotypic expression is covered up (masked) by its own dominant allele.

- **Recessive** tending to recede; (in genetics).

- **Recombinant DNA (r-DNA)** A strand or DNA synthesized in the laboratory by splicing together selected parts of DNA strands from different organic species or by adding a selected part to an existing DNA strand.

■ **Recombination** A new combination of phenotypes in offspring by mating parents with different phenotypes.

■ **Rectified** Refind.

■ **Rectum** commences on a level with the anterior opening of the pelvis and extends to the anus.

■ **Red meat** Meat that is red when raw.

■ **Red water** also called Bacillary Hemoglobinuria. *Clostridium haemolyticum* is the cause.

■ **Red worms** The common name for Strongyles. These can cause severe anaemia and debility.

■ **Reduction disease** Metabolic diseases attributable to the imbalance between rate of input of dietary nutrients and output of production.

■ **Reflex** An involuntary response to a stimulus.

■ **Reflex** action is one of the simplest forms of activity of the nervous system.

■ **Refract** to cause to deviate.

■ **Refraction** The act or process of refracting.

■ **Regeneration** Regaining of tissues or organs lost or healing of the wounds.

■ **Region** Plane area with more or less definite boundaries.

■ **Regional anesthesia** It is the loss of sensation in a larger, area of the body.

■ **Rehabilitation** Restoration to useful activity of persons with physical or other disability.

■ **Relapse** Reoccurence.

■ **Remedy** Anything that cures or palliates disease.

■ **Ren** Hypermobile kidney.

■ **Renal** Relating to the kidney.

■ **Renin** A proteolytic enzyme obtained from a cell's stomach that forms curd from milk.

■ **Rennet** A proteolytic enzyme, rein, used in cheese making.

■ **Repeatability** The tendency for an individual to repeat its performance, measured as an intra-class correlation based on repeated records of the same animal.

■ **Reproductive cycle** Also sexual cycle, oestrus cycle. Cyclical changes in animal behaviour reproductive functions of a mature female, comprising periods of pro-estrus, oestrus, metoes-trus and dioestrus.

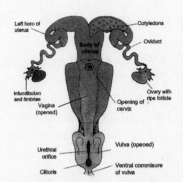

Labels:
Left horn of uterus
Cotyledons
Body of uterus
Oviduct
Infundibulum and fimbriae
Vagina (opened)
Opening of cervix
Ovary with ripe follicle
Urethral orifice
Vulva (opened)
Clitoris
Ventral commisure of vulva

REPRODUCTIVE SYSTEM

- **Reserve** to hold back for future use.

- **Reservoir** Storage place or cavity.

- **Residual** Remaining or left behind.

- **Residue** Remainder; that remaining after removal of other substances.

- **Resonant** Giving an intense, rich sound on percussion.

- **Respiratory system** Respiratory system consists of nose, pharynx, larynx, trachea, bronchi and lung.

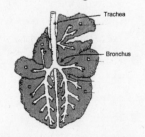

Labels:
Trachea
Bronchus

RESPIRATORY SYSTEM

- **Response** Any action or change of condition evoked by a stimulus.

- **Retained placenta** A placenta that is not expelled, or vioded, at parturition.

- **Retardation** delay; hindrance; delayed development.

- **Rete testis** A system of collection tubules draining the seminiferous tubules.

- **Retention** the process of holding back or keeping in position.

- **Reticulocyte** Any non-nucleated cell of the erythrocytic series containing RNA, which when suppravitally stained with new methliene blue or brilliant crystyl blue will have discernible granules or a diffuse network of fibrils.

- **Reticulum** This pyriform sac is the smallest of all other compartments and situated between the diaphragm and liver in front and dorsal sac of rumen and omasum behind.

- **Retina** Innermost of the three layers of vertebrate eye, except in front; it is sensitive to light.

■ **Reticulo-endothelial system**
A widely spread network of
body cells concerned with
blood cell formation, bile
formation and engulfing or
trapping of foreign materials,
which includes cells of bone
marrow, lymph, spleen, and
liver.

■ **Retro** is a prefix signifying
behind or turned backward.

■ **Reversible reaction** A chemical reaction in which the
end products can readily
revert to the original molecules.

■ **Rh** Symbol for Rhesus factor
(blood)

■ **Rheumatism** A general term
indicating diseases of muscles, tendons, joints, bones
or nerves resulting in pain
and disability.

■ **Rhin(o)** nose; nose-like
structure.

■ **Rhodopsion** A conjugated
protein present in the rods of
retina which is responsible
for dim light vision.

■ **Rhinitis** Inflammation of
mucous membrane of nasal
cavity.

■ **Rhythm** Measured movement; the recurrence of an
action or function at regular
intervals.

■ **Riboflavin** B_2 Vitamin that
functions as a flavoprotein.

■ **Ribosomes** are granules containing RNA.

■ **Ribs** These are curved elongated bones arranged one
after another from either side
of the vertebral column and
form the thoracic cage.

■ **Rice polish** The material
obtained during the polish-
ing of rice kernels after initial removal of hulls and
bran.

■ **Rickettsia** The generic name
for a group of minute microorganisms which may be said
to be intermediate between
the smallest bacteria and the
viruses.

■ **Rickets** Disease of young
one's characterised by inadequate deposition of Ca salts
in the growing bone.

■ **Ridgling (rigling)** Any male
animal whose testicles fail to
descend into the scrotum.
Also called a cryptochid.

■ **Rifamycin** An antibiotic
that inhibits bacterial RNA
synthesis.

■ **Right atrium** Thin walled
muscular chamber of heart is
smaller than the left and

receives venous blood from the body.

- **Right ventricle** It forms the right and cranial part of the heart.

- **Rigor mortis** The stiffening or hardening of muscles soon after death.

- **Rim** Border or edge.

- **Ring** Any annular or circular organ or area.

- **Rinderpest** Rinderpest is an acute, highly contagious disease of ruminants and swine caused by a virus and characterized by high fever and focal, erosive lesions confined largely to the mucosa of the digestive tract.

- **Ring bone** Exostosis on 1st and 2nd phalynx.

- **Ringworm** Ringworm is caused by the invasion of the keratinized epithelial cells and hair fibres by dermatophytes.

- **Ripened cream** Butter made from cream that has been ripened by the addition of a starter culture.

- **RO** Reverse osmosis.

- **Roan** A mixture of red and white hair in the coat of shorthorns. In horses, it is a mixture of dark hairs (any color) with white hairs.

- **Roaring** Respiratory noise produced due to paralysis of vocal cords.

- **Roasting** Roasting is accomplished by passing the grain through a flame or heating it to the desired temperature in some form of an oven for a period of time, resulting in some expansion of the grain.

- **Rodenticides** Drugs used to kill rodents.

- **Rolled** Compressed into flat particles by having been passed between rollers.

- **Ropy milk** Also known as stringy milk. Such milk, when poured, has a rope-like form.

- **Rot** Decay; disease of sheep.

- **Rotavirus** Any of a group of double-standard RNA viruses.

- **Roughage** A coarse feeding stuff generally high in fibre but low in its percentage of digestible matter as contrasted with that of concentrates. Hay, fodder and straw are common roughages.

- **Rubefacients** are a class of blistering agents that are mild in character.

- **Rudiment** Vestigial organ.
- **Rudimentary** Imperfectly developed; vestigial.
- **Rumen** The first and the largest of the four compartments which form the stomach of a ruminant ; contains a large number of organisms which play an essential role in ruminant nutrition.

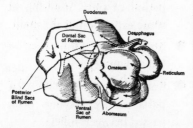

RUMEN OF COW

- **Rumenotoric Action** Agents which bring about tone and contractions of rumen.
- **Ruminal stasis** Ruminal contractions are feeble or nil which bring about stasis of rumen.
- **Ruminal** Tympany (Bloat) Over-distension of the rumen and reticulum with the gases of fermentation, either mixed with or separated from the fluid and solid ingesta.
- **Ruminant** Cud chewing animal, having four distinct compartments of stomach.
- **Rumination** (chewing the cud) Act of regurgitating food from rumen for chewing and mixing with saliva before returning it to the rumen.
- **Rut** The period or season of heightened sexual activity in some male mammals, coinciding with estrus in females.
- **Rutation** The process of turning around an axis.
- **Rye bran** The coarse outer covering of the rye kernel as removed in the usual processes, other than scouring.

❏

S/s

■ **s.i.d** once in a day

■ **s.o.s.** if necessary

■ **Sacral vertebra** Vertebra of tetrapods, which articulates hip region with ilia of hip-girdle.

■ **Sacrum** This bone is formed by the fusion of five sacral vertebrae in cow and in horse.

■ **Saggital** Shaped like an arrow.

■ **Saggital plane** Parallel to median plane.

■ **Salicylates** Drugs that have been derivatives of salicylic acid.

■ **Saliva** Secretion of salivary glands.

■ **Salivary glands** Three pairs of glands in the mouth which secrete saliva.

■ **Salk vaccine** A preparation of a formalin-inactivated polio virus that is injected.

■ **Salmonella** A genus of gram-negative bacteria.

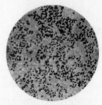

SALMONELLA

■ **Salmonellosis** or Paratyphoid Salmonellosis is a disease of all animal species caused by a number of different species of salmonellae manifested clinically by a peracute septicaemia, acute enteritis or a chronic enteritis.

■ **Salping(o)** Tube (Eustachian tube or uterine tube).

■ **Salpingitis** Inflammation of fallopian tube.

■ **Salt** A substance that dissolves in water to cations and anions, neither of which is H+ or OH-.

■ **Salt balance** In milk the ratio between calcium plus magnesium ions to phosphate plus citrate ions.

■ **Salty milk** Mastitis and late lactation, produce changes resulting in a decrease in the lactose and an increase in the salt content.

■ **Sanitation** Removal of microbes from eating utensils and food preparation areas.

■ **Sanitization** Use of methods and materials to preserve or restore hygienic quality.

■ **Sanitizing** Destroy pathogenic organisms but does not ensure complete removal.

■ **Sapremia** Condition which results from the absorption of the end-products irrigation is called sapremia.

■ **Saprophyte** An organism that obtains its nutrients from dead organic maatter.

■ **Saprophytic bacteria** Those which live on dead matter.

■ **Sarco** is a prefix signifying flesh or fleshy.

■ **Sarcoma** A cancer of fleshy, nonepithelial tissue or connective tissue.

■ **Sarcoptic Mange** Sarcoptic mange occurs in all species causing a severe itching dermatitis.

■ **Satellitosis** Accumulation of glial cells around the degenerating neuron.

■ **Scab** The crust which forms on superficial injured areas, is composed of fibrin.

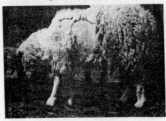

SHEEP SCAB

■ **Scabies** A parasitic skin disease caused by the itch mite. Highly contagious.

■ **Scald** Inflammation between the digits of young sheep, causing acute lameness.

■ **Scapula** It is a flat triangular bone situated at the craniolateral aspect of the thorax.

■ **Scar** Cicatrix ; a mark remaining after the healing of a wound.

■ **Schistosomiasis** Infestation with *Schistosoma* worms or flukes.

■ **Schizogony** The process of multiple fission, in which one organism divides to produce many daughter cells.

■ **Schizont** A malarial parasite of the asexual generation.

■ **Sciatica** means pain connected with the sciatic nerve which runs down the thigh.

■ **Science** The systematic observation of natural phenomena for the purpose of discovering laws governing those phenomena.

■ **Sclera** is the outermost hard fibrous coat of the eye.

■ **Sclerosis** Word used in pathology to describe abnormal hardening or fibrosis of a tissue.

■ **Scolex** The head of a tape-worm, containing suckers and possibly hooks.

■ **Score card** A numerical standard of excellence with definite values assigned for different aspects; a basis for judgement of a product or an animal.

■ **Scirrhous cord** Excessive granulation tissue formed on the stump of severed spermatic cord usually due to infection with staphylococci.

■ **Screen** A structure resembling a curtain or partition, used as a protection or shield.

■ **Screw-worm flies** These belong to the sub-family *Calliphorinae*, includes the grenbottles, bluebottles, and the flies cause 'Strike'.

■ **Scrotum** The thin sac containing the testes.

■ **Scurs** Rudimentary horns which are not attached to the bony part of the head.

■ **Scurvey** A pathological condition due to lack of vitamin C. Gums bleed.

■ **Seat worm** is another name for the threadworm or oxyuris.

■ **Sebaceous gland** Epidermal skin gland of mammals, embedded in dermis, nearly always opening into a hair follicle, secreting fatty substance (sebum).

■ **Seborrhoea** Seborrhoea is an excessive secretion of sebum on to the skin surface.

■ **Second filial generation** The generation following the first filial (F1) generation. It is referred to as the F2 generation.

■ **Secondary infection** An infection caused by an opportunistic pathogen after a primary infection has weakened the host's defenses.

■ **Secretion** The passage of material produced by a cell from the inside to the outside of its plasma membrane.

■ **Section** An act of cutting.

■ **Sectomy** Words ending in this way mean surgical removal of.

■ **Sediment** A precipitate, especially that formed spontaneously.

■ **Sedative drugs** Refers to the drugs which are used to sedate, that is to calm, anxious and restless patients without making sleep.

- **Sediment test** A simple, rapid and quantitative test to find gross impurities and dirt in milk due to unhygienic production, storage and transportation.

- **Seedstock herd** Herd maintained for producing breeding animals for commercial purpose.

- **Segment** A demarcated portion of a whole.

- **Segregation of genes** Genes occur in body cells in pairs but in sex cells in half pairs. Thus a gene of a pair in the individual segregates (separates) from its mate when sex cells are produced.

- **Selection** Choosing animals to produce progenies which will contribute to next generation.

- **Selenium** Sodium selenate is used by horticulturists as an insectcide.

- **Semen** Sperms together with secretions of various accessory glands.

- **Seminal vesicle** These are two lobulated elongated glands situated below the rectum.

- **Seminiferous** tubules Minute tubules making up

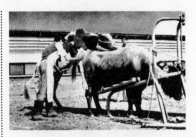

SEMEN COLLECTION

the major portion of the testicle and which produce the sperm or male sex cells from a layer of spermatogonia cells lining the tubules.

- **Semisynthetic** produced by chemical manipulation of naturally occurring substances.

- **Senna** A standardised preparation of this household laxative recommended in treating or preventing constipation.

- **Sensation** An impression produced by impulses covered by an afferent nerve to the sensorium.

- **Sensitisation** is the prdouction of a certain degree of anaphylaxis by a particular protein, vaccine, antibiotic, etc.

- **Sensory** Pertaining to sensation.

■ **Separator** It is a mechanical device to separate milk fat from serum (separated milk).

■ **Sepsis** The presence of unwanted bacteria.

■ **Septic tank** A tank, built into the ground, in which waste water is treated by primary treatment.

■ **Septicemia** A condition characterized by the multiplication of bacteria in the blood.

■ **Septum** A crosswall dividing two parts.

■ **Sequestrum** A fragment of bone that has become necrotic and has separated from normal healthy bone.

■ **Sera** Plural of serum.

■ **Series** A group or succession of events, objects.

■ **Serious** Grave, staid.

■ **Serology** The branch of immunology concerned with the study of antigen-antibody reactions in vitro.

■ **Serum** The fluid that remains after blood clots.

■ **Service** The act of natural breeding in cattle.

■ **Service** period Time between the date of calving and the date of conception.

■ **Severe** Harsh, stern.

■ **Sex-chromosomes** Chromosomes which are particularly connected with the determination of sex.

■ **Sex-limited** characteristics Expressed in only one sex i.e. milk production.

■ **Sheath** The long tube in which the penis moves at the time of collecting semen for use in artificial insemination.

■ **Sheep Ked** (*Melophagus ovinus*) is a wingless blood-sucking parasite.

■ **Sheep pox and Goat pox** In sheep pox typical pox lesions occur particularly under the tail. A malignant form with a general distribution of lesions occurs in lambs caused by virus.

■ **Sheet** An oblong piece of cotton, linen, etc. for a bed covering.

■ **Shield** Any protecting structure.

■ **Shift** A change or deviation.

■ **Shift to left** An increase in the immature forms of the granulocytic series in the blood.

■ **Shift to right** An increase in the percent of older cells (hypersegmentation).

■ **Shigella** Genus of gram-negative.

■ **Shivering** is a nervous disease of horses, characterised by spasmodic contractions of certain groups of muscles, particularly in the hindquararaters and tail.

■ **Shock** Condition of collapse which may follow severe injury, surgical operations, haemorrhage and other conditions.

■ **Shorts** A by-product of flour milling consisting of a mixture of small particles of bran and germ, the aleurone layer, and coarse flour.

■ **Shoulder** joint Ball and socket joint, cavity of scapula and head of humerus.

■ **Shunt** to turn to one side; to bypass.

■ **Sialoliths** Concretions in the excretory ducts of parotid, sublingual and submaxillary salivary glands.

■ **Sib** The brother or sister of an individual.

■ **Side-effects** The side-effects of a drug are those prdouced in addition to that for which purpose the drug is given.

■ **Sign** Indication of the existence of something; any objective evidence of a disease.

■ **Signa** The signa (Sig. or S.) consists of instructions for administration of the medicine.

■ **Signs** Changes due to a disease that a physician can observe and measure.

■ **Silage** Silage is a fermented feed resulting from the storage of high moisture crops, usually green forages, under anaerobic conditions in a structure known as a silo.

■ **Silicon** A non-metallic element. Silicon is essential for growth, and is found mainly in connective tissue.

■ **Silo** Under or above ground structure used for preserving feed or grains.

■ **Sinus** A hollow or cavity, especially the nasal sinuses.

■ **Sire** Male parent.

■ **Skeleton** It can be defined as a hard framework of the body, which supports soft structures. This is composed of bones, cartilages and ligaments.

■ **Skewbald** A spotted horse whose dark spots are any other color but black.

■ **Skin** Covering of the body.

■ **Skull** is the collection of flat and irregularly shaped bones, which protects the brain and forms the skeleton of the face.

■ **Sleeper** syndrome Thromboembolic meningo-encephalitis.

■ **Slipped tendon** (Perosis) A condition in chickens due to deficiency of manganese characterized by displacement of tendon and an inability for the leg to support the birds weight.

■ **Slings** A device whereby a large animal may be kept in the standing position for long periods without becoming completely exhausted.

■ **Slough** means a dead part separated by natural processes from the rest of the living body.

■ **Slurry** is the liquid mixture of urine and faeces.

■ **Smear** A thin film of material on a slide.

■ **Smell** The sense of smell is situated in the nasal mucous membrane, and in the nerve centres of the brain which are connected with the nasal mucosa by the olfactory nerves.

■ **Smooth ER** Endoplasmic reticulum without ribosomes.

■ **Smooth** Plain or even.

■ **Sneezing** is a sudden expulsion of air through the nostrils, designed to expel irritating materials from the upper air passages; the vocal cords being kept shut.

■ **Snoaring** Respiratory noise which is produced due to pharyngeal obstruction.

■ **Snout** It is formed by the apex of the nose and the upper lip.

■ **Sodium** is a metal whose salts are white, crystalline, and very soluble in water.

■ **Sodium monofluoroacetate** Also known as '1080', this is a rodenticide.

■ **Soft curd milk** This may be defined as milk which, when treated with rennet, does not give a firm clot.

■ **Soggy** A texture defect in ice cream due to lack of proper whipping or incorporation of air.

■ **Solar** Pertaining to the sun.

■ **Sole** The sole is slightly concave and placed at the ground surface of the hoof.

- **Solubility** The ability to be dissolved, usually in water.
- **Solute** A substance dissolved in another substance.
- **Solvent** A dissolving medium.
- **Somatic** Refers to body cells or tissues. All the cells belonging to the body except germ cells.
- **Sorbet** Synonym of sherbet; a fruit-flavoured ice, typically served between courses as palate refresher.
- **Sorbic acid** A permitted preservative used in cheese to the extent of 0.1 per cent, either as such or as its calcium, potassium and sodium salts.
- **Sore throat** is a popular term for laryngitis or pharyngitis. Often present during catarrh, strangles, influenza.
- **Sorrel** A coat color of horses that includes the red shades of chestnut, or yellowish brown.
- **S.O.S.** si o'pus sit (if necessary)
- **Sow** A breeding female pig after the first litter.
- **Soyabean milk** Milky fluid prepared from soyabeans.

- **Spasm** A sudden, violent, involuntary muscular contraction.
- **Spasmodic** of the nature of a spasm; occurring in spasms.
- **Spasmolytics** Agents which control spasms.
- **Spastic** is a term applied to any condition showing a tendency to spasm, such as 'spastic gait'.
- **Spavin** Exostosis on the medial portion of distal tarsal bones.
- **Spay** To remove the ovaries.
- **Spaying** is the term commonly used for the removal of the ovaries in the female.
- **Specialist** A physician whose practice is limited to a particular branch of medicine or surgery, especially one.
- **Species** A group of animals or plants which have in common, one or more distinctive characters by which they may be differentiated from other such groups.
- **Specific** is a term used in various ways. It is applied to remedies that have a definite curative effect on certain diseases.

- **Specimen** A small sample or part taken to show the nature of the whole,

- **Speculum** is an instrument designed to aid the examination of the various openings of the body surface.

- **Speech** The expression of thoughts and ideas by vocal sounds.

- **Spermatic cord** It extends from the internal abdominal ring of the inguinal canal to the upper end of the corresponding testis.

- **Spermatogenesis** The process by which sperm cells are formed in the testes of the male (gametogenesis in the male).

- **Spermatozoa or sperms** Are the motile male sex cells which having matured in the epidermis are ejaculated at orgasm and are normally capable of fertilizing the ovum or egg.

- **Spermicidal agents** Refer to agents that are able to kill spermatozoa or that hasten their degeneration by impeding their passage through the cervical canal.

- **Sphere** A ball or globe.

- **Sphero** Round; a sphere.

- **Spheroplast** A Gram-negative bacterium treated to damage the cell wall, resulting in a spherical cell.

- **Sphincter** A circular muscle which surrounds the opening from an organ, prevents the escape of the contents of the organ.

- **Sphygmograph** is an instrument used for recording the pulse.

- **Spinal column** the chain of bones reaching from the base of the skull along the neck and back to the tip of the tail, is composed of the vertebrae.

- **Spinal cord** This is a thick cylindrical structure situated in the vertebral column and lies loosely by its covering. It extends from the foramen magnum to the middle of the sacrum.

- **Spiral** Winding like the thread of a screw.

- **Spirilla** The more loosely curved cells are known as spirilla.

- **Spirits** These are alcoholic solutions of volatile drugs.

- **Spirochaetes** Spirochaetes are microorganisms which are slender and spiral in shape, motile by means of a flexuous motion and they multiply by transverse fission.

■ **Splanchnology** Study of the viscereal organs of different systems.

■ **Spleen** Spleen is a hemolymph organ situated obliquely downward and left part of the abdomen between the left face of the rumen and diaphragm.

■ **Splenectomy** Surgical removal of the spleen.

■ **Splint** Exostosis of ends of metacarpal or metatarsal bones.

■ **Splint** A rigid or flexible appliance for fixation of displaced or movable parts.

■ **Spondyl(o)** Vertebra.

■ **Spondylitis** Inflammation of vertebrae.

■ **Spondylosis** Loosening or breaking down of a vertebra.

■ **Spongiosis** Intercellular oedema of epidermis.

■ **Sporadic disease** A disease that occurs occasionally in a population.

■ **Spore** A vegetative or reproductive body of microscopic size produced by bacteria and fungi.

■ **Sporotrichosis** Sportotrichosis is a contagious disease of horses characterized by the development of cutaneous nodules and ulcers on the limbs and may or may not be accompanied by lymphangitis.

■ **Sporulation** The process of spore formation.

■ **Sprains** involve the wrenching of a joint, often with the simultaneous tearing of a ligament.

■ **Sprays** consisting of antiparasitic dressings, are sometimes used in the treatment of mange.

■ **Spray drying** A process of drying milk–whole, condensed, skim or butter–by spraying into chamber of heated air, ;the temperature ranging from 25°F to 300°F.

■ **Spreads** Dairy spreads are preparations resembling very soft cheese and butter, prepared from any or all of the following milk and whey solids, cheese (various), fats (various), emulsifying agents, vegetable and plant extracts or powder, seasoning, condiments and colouring matter.

■ **Stablilzers** Substances which stabilize milk against heat coagulation, e.g. citric acid, citrates, phosphates, carbonates, bicarbonates.

■ **Stables** Ideal house for horse keeping.

■ **Stag** A male animal castrated late in life so that it still retains some of the secondary sex characteristics of the mature, intact male.

■ **Staitness** Accumulation of ceroid in the tissues giving yellowish brown colouration.

■ **Stallion** A mature, intact male horse.

■ **Standard** Something established as a measure or model to which other similar things should conform.

■ **Staphylococci** Gram positive bacterium which appears as grapelike cluster of spherical cells under the microscope.

■ **Star-gazing syndrome** Thiamine deficiency in birds.

■ **Starter culture** Microbial cultures producing lactic acid enzymes and other desired changes in milk and milk products.

■ **Starting milk** Removal of coarse particles from milk by passing it through a number of materials as cheese cloth, cotton pad, etc.

■ **Starvation** Complete deprivation of food.

■ **Stassanisation** A method of pasteurization of milk in a tubular heat-exchanger, consisting of these concentric tubes.

■ **Stat** At once.

■ **State** Condition or situation.

■ **Status** condition or state.

■ **Staxis** Hemorrhage.

■ **Steam flaking** Grain is subjected to high moisture steam for a sufficient time to raise the water content to 18-20 per cent and the grain is then rolled to produce a rather flat flake.

■ **Steatitis** A general increase in the fatty constituents of the body.

■ **Steer** Male calf castrated before sexual maturity.

■ **Steno** Narrows; contracted.

■ **Stenosis** is any unnatural narrowing of a passage or orifice of the body.

■ **Sterile** In bacteriology, free from all living organisms.

In animal husbandry, incapable of producing offspring.

■ **Sterility** Lacking the power to produce offspring.

■ **Sterilization** A process of freeing a commodity of living microorganisms.

■ **Sternum** (Breast bone) It is long plate of osteo-cartilagenous structure placed at the midline of the floor of the thoracic cavity.

■ **Steroids** A specific group of chemical substances, including cholesterol and hormones.

■ **Sterol** A lipid alcohol found in the plasma membranes of fungi and Mycoplasma.

■ **Stethoscope** An instrument for performing mediate auscultation.

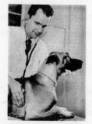

STETHOSCOPE

■ **Stiff lamb disease** Syn. White muscle disease. Caused by vitamin E deficiency.

■ **Stifle** Joint It is a complex joint comprises of two articulations—1) Femoro-patellar—Trochlea of femur and articular surface of pattela. 2) Femoro Tibial—Condyles of femur and proximal end of tibia.

■ **Stilboestrol** This is an oestrogen used both therapeutically and as a growth promoter in food animal.

■ **Stillbirth** Expulsion of dead foetus at full term.

■ **Stimulation** Increases the activity of specialized cells.

■ **Stimulus** Anything which excites functional activity in an organ or part.

■ **Stimulants** Heart stimulants include caffeine, digitalis, strychnine, coramine.

■ **Stimulate** To excite functional activity in a party.

■ **Sting** Injury due to a biotoxin introduced into an individual or by bites.

■ **Stirk** A young bull or cow less than two years old.

■ **Stitching** Suturing

■ **Stomach** The main digestive organ, has four compartments in ruminants–rumen, reticulum, omasum and abomasum.

- **Stomach-tube** is a rubber tube from 9 to 10 ft long for horses and cattle, used for introducing into the stomach relieving tympany.

- **Stomat (o)** Mouth.

- **Stomatitis** Stomatitis is inflammation of the oral mucosa.

- **Stover** Mature cured stalks of grain from which the ears have been removed, used as feed.

- **Strain** To overexercise; to use to an extreme and harmful degree.

- **Strain** A group of cells derived from a single cell.

- **Strangles** Strangles is an acute disease of horses caused by infection with *Streptococcus equi*. It is characterized by inflammation of the upper respiratory tract and abscessation in the adjacent lymph nodes.

- **Strangulation** Term applied to the stoppage of the circulation.

- **Straws** The part of the mature plants remaining after the removal of grains by thrashing or combing.

- **Strepto** Twisted.

- **Streptococcus** A microorganism which under the microscope has much the appearance of string beads.

- **Streptobacilli** Rods that remain attached in chains after cell division.

- **Streptomycin** Antibiotics derived from sugar.

- **Stress** Forcibly exerted influence; pressure. A physical, chemical or emotional factor along with management errors that cause physiological or mental tension and may be a contributory factor towards lower production and disease causation.

- **Stricture** means a narrowing of one of the natural passages of the body, such as the gullet, bowel, or urethra.

- **Stridor** Harsh sound in breathing caused by air passing through obstructed air passages.

- **Stringhalt** is the sudden snatching up of one or both hind-legs of the horse when walking.

- **Strip** The last milk taken out of udder after the bulk of milk is drawn.

- **Stroke** A sudden severe attack.

- **Strongyles** Red worms.
- **Struck** Disease caused by *Clostridium perfringens* type C.
- **Strychnine** is one of the two chief alkaloids of the seed of *Strychnos nux vomica*. Strychnine itself is a white crystalline substance bitter.
- **Stunted** Arrest in growth or development.
- **Sty** A small, hard, red swelling on the edge of the eyelid.
- **Sub** Under; near; almost; moderately.
- **Subacute disease** A disease with symptoms between acute and chronic.
- **Subclinical** infection An infection that does not cause a noticeable illness.
- **Subcutaneous** Inoculation just beneath the skin is the most common.
- **Subconscious** Imperfectly or partially conscious.
- **Sublimation** the conversion of a solid directly into the gaseous state.
- **Sublingual** Beneath the tongue.
- **Sublingualadministration** Administration, usually in tablet form, under the tongue.

- **Substance** Material constituting and organ or body.
- **Substrate** The substance acted upon by the enzyme is called a substrate.
- **Succulent** Soft, pliable, juicy feed relatively low in fibre content and easily digestible.
- **Suck** To draw milk directly into mouth by creasing vaccum with muscles of lips.
- **Sufficient** Adequate, enough.
- **Suffocation** Interruption to breathing.
- **Suitable** Fit, appropriate.
- **Sulfaguandine** An antibacterial sulfonamide.
- **Sulfamerazine** An antibacterial sulfonamide.
- **Sulfamethizole** An antibacterial sulfonamide.
- **Sulfa drugs** Any synthetic chemotherapeutic agent containing sulfur and nitrogen.
- **Sulfanilamide** A potent antibacterial compound.
- **Sulfonamide** The chemical group SO_2NH_2.
- **Sulfurated** Combined or charged with sulfur.
- **Sulphur** is a non-metallic element which is procurable

in several different allotropic forms.

■ **Sulphur dioxide** A poisonous gas which is a constituent of Diesel engine exhaust fumes.

■ **Summer mastitis** Mastitis of non-lacatating animals caused by *Corynebacterium pyogenes*.

■ **Summer sores** in horses are caused by infective *Hebronema* larvae deposited in wounds by stable or house flies.

■ **Sunstroke** or Heatstroke.

■ **Superfetation** Two pregnancies at different times in the same gestation period of the female.

■ **Super** is a prefix signifying above or implying excess.

■ **Superficial** Situated on or near the surface. Close to surface.

■ **Superfoundation** When offspring from 2 or 3 sexes are present e.g. Bitches (different phenotype character).

■ **Superinfection** (1) Growth of the target pathogen that has developed resistance to the antimicrobial drug being used. (2) Growth of an opportunistic pathogen.

■ **Superior** Situated above; or directed upward.

■ **Supersonic** Traveling faster than the speed of sound.

■ **Superovulation** The stimulation of multiple ovulation with fertility drugs.

■ **Supplement** A semi-concentrated source of one or more nutrients used to enhance the nutritional adequacy of a daily ration or a complete ration mixture.

■ **Suppositories** These are solid drug forms intended for conveyance of drugs into body cavities. They are inserted into the rectum, vagina, and urethra.

■ **Suppuration** The formation of pus.

■ **Supravital** staining Staining of cells with a stain of low toxicity that will not cause death of the living cells, so that vital and functional process may be studied in the cells.

■ **Supra** Above; over.

■ **Surface** The outer part or external aspect of an object.

■ **Surfactants** Surface active agents that are able to reduce surface tension.

■ **Surgery** That branch of medicine which treats diseases, and deformities by manual or operative methods.

- **Surra** is a disease of most economic importance in camels and horses, can affect domestic animals and is caused by a blood protozoan.

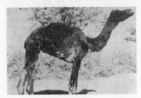

SURRA

- **Susceptible** Readily affected or acted upon; lacking immunity or resistance.

- **Susceptibility** The lack of resistance to a disease.

- **Suture** is the name given either to the close union between two adjacent edges or to a series of stitches by which a wound is closed.

- **Swabs** Swabs are used for sampling mucus, etc., for diagnostic purposes.

- **Swallowing** Swallowing is a complex act governed by reflexes and includes closure of all exits from pharynx, creation of pressure to force substance into the oesophagus and involuntarily to stomach.

- **Swayback** is a disease of new born and young lambs, characterised by progressive cerebral demyelination, which results in paralysis and often death.

- **Sweet** In dairying this term means non-acid or non-soured or non-ripened, as also free from taint.

- **Sweet cream** Butter made from cream containing not mor than 0.2 per cent acid at any time.

- **Swine influenza** Swine influenza is a viral, highly contagious disease of pigs characterized clinically by fever and signs of respiratory involvement.

- **Swine pox** Swine pox is usually a benign disease characterized by the appearance of typical pox lesions on the ventral abdomen caused by virus.

- **Swine dysentery** characterised by haemorrhagic enteritis.

- **Swine erysipelas** is an infectious disease of pigs and characterised by high fever, reddish or purplish spots on the skin, haemmorhage on to the surfaces of certain the internal organs in acute cases.

■ **Swine fever** hog cholera, pig tyhphoid, is highly infectious and contagious disease of pigs. The cause is a virus, associated with *Salmonella, Pasteurella* and *Actinomyces*.

■ **Swirl** Hair on an animal that grows in opposite directions (swirl) to the rest of the hair on the body.

■ **Sylene** dimethylbenzene, CaH_{10}. used an a solvent in microscopy.

■ **Syn** is a prefix signifying union.

■ **Synchronisation of oestrus** Controlled breeding by bringing group of animals to heat.

■ **Symbiosis** The living together of two different organisms.

■ **Sympathetic system** This system is composed of two ganglionated sympathetic trunks extending along each of the vertebral column.

■ **Symptom** A change in body function that is felt by a patient as a result of a disease.

■ **Synapse** This is the junction where one neuron ends and other neuron begins.

■ **Synapsis** The coming together of paired chromosomes during the first meiotic division.

■ **Syndesmology** Study of Joints.

■ **Syndrome** A set of symptoms occurring together; the sum of signs of any morbid state; a symptom complex.

■ **Synergism** The principle whereby the effectiveness of two drugs used simultaneously is greater than that of either drug used alone.

■ **Synergistic action** Refers to a drug action that increases the effect produced by another drug.

■ **Synovial fluid** It is a lubricant fluid secreted by the synovial membrane.

■ **Synovial joints** These joints are formed by articular cartilages, joint capsule and ligaments.

■ **Synovial membrane** It is a thin membrane which lines the joint cavity, synovial bursa and synovial tendon sheath.

■ **Synthetic drugs** Drugs produced in the chemical laboratory in a more pure state for the prevention, treatment, and alleviation of disease.

- **Synthetic milk** Artificial milk obtained from non-dairy sources.

- **Synthesis** Creation of a compound by union of elements composing it, done artificially or as a result of natural processes.

- **Syringe** A device of plastic, glass, steel.

- **Systole** means the contraction of the heart as opposed to the resting phase is called 'diastole'.

- **Systematic Bacteriology** Embraces the classification and nomenclature of bacteria.

- **Systemic (generalized) function** An infection throughout the body.

- **Systemic Anatomy** Study of the structures of the body system-wise.

❏

- **T cell** A type of lymphocyte, which develops from a stem cell processed in the thymus gland, that is responsible for cell-mediated immunity.

- **t.i.d.** 3 times a day

- **tab** tablet

- **Tablets** Tablets are made by compressing powders mechanically into small discoid shapes.

- **Tachycardia** Increased heart rate.

- **Tachyphagia** Rapid eating

- **Taenia** A tapeworm.

- **Talfan disease** Viral encephalomyelitis of pigs, Teschen disease.

- **Tallowiness** A flavour defect in butter due to oxidation of unsaturated fatty acid, catalysed by traces of copper and oxidizing enzymes.

- **T-antigen** An antigen in the nucleus of a tumor cell.

- **Tannin or Tanic acid** is a noncrystallisable white or pale-yellowish powder, which is very soluble in water prepared from oak-galls. Tannin is also found in strong tea or coffee.

- **Tapping** is the popular name for the withdrawal of fluid from body cavities, or the subcutaneous tissues of the body.

- **Tapeworm** A flatworm belonging to the class Cestoda.

- **Tapioca chips** Thin sliced pieces of tapioca tubes in dried condition.

- **Tar** is the thick, oily, strong-smelling, black liquid which is obtained by distillation from coal and wood.

- **Tarsal bones** There are five tarsal bones and the lateral. These short bones are situated between the distal end of tibia and proximal ends of metatarsal bones to form hock joint.

- **Tarsus** The ankle or corresponding part of the hindlimb.

- **Tartar** emetic is also called 'tartrated antimony', or antimony potassium tartrate, white crystalline substance, once popular as a medicine. Specific in Leishmaniasis is also used in the treatment of certain forms of trypanoso-miasis.

■ **Taste** Sense organs for taste buds located on the surface of the tongue.

■ **Taste bud** A small sense organ in most vertebrates, specialized for the detection of taste.

■ **Tattooing** This is done, by means of a special pair of forceps or indelible ink, for the purpose of identifying farm live-stock.

■ **Taxonomy** The science of classification.

■ **TDN** Abbreviation for total digestible nutrients.

■ **Teat** The protuberance on the udder through which milk is drawn from a mammal.

■ **Teeth** Teeth are the hardest structures in the body. They are implanted into the alveolar sockets of the upper and lower jaw bones.

■ **Tele** Far at a distance.

■ **Telophase** The fourth stage of mitosis. It is characaterised by an elongation of the chromosomes, the disappearance of the spindle fibers, and the reorganization of the nuclear membrane.

■ **Temporary** Short, brief.

■ **Temple** The lateral region on either side of the head.

■ **Tendon** A thick strand or sheet of tissue that attaches a muscle to a bone.

■ **Tenotomy** means an operation in which one or more tendons are severed by a surgical incision.

■ **Teratogen** A substance which is able to deform the fetus in the womb and so induce birth defects.

■ **Terratogenicity** Abnormalities produced in the offspring of an animal by taking some material by the mother during pregnancy.

■ **Terramycin** Antibiotic which was isolated in 1950 from *Streptomyces rimosus.* (*Oxytetracycline*)

■ **Teschen diseae** See Talfan disease.

■ **Test cross** A mating test to determine if an individual is a carrier of a recessive gene.

■ **Testicle** The organ of the male animal which produces and stores the male sex cell as well as producing testoterone, the male hormone.

■ **Testis** (testicide) The reproductive organ in male animals in which spermatozoa are produced.

■ **Testosterone** The 'male' hormone produced by the interstitial cells in the testicle and which causes the male to develop the typical male characteristics.

■ **Tetanus** Tetanus is a highly fatal, infectious disease of all species of domestic animals caused by the toxin of *Clostridium tetani*. It is characterized clinically by hyperaesthesia, tetany and convulsions.

■ **Tetany** Condition of muscular hyperexcitability in which mild stimuli produce cramps and spasms. Found in parathyroid deficiency and alkalosis.

■ **Tetra** Four.

■ **Tetramisole** An anthelmintic for use against gastrointestinal roundworms and lungworms.

■ **Tetracycline** Broad-spectrum antibiotics that interfere with protein synthesis.

■ **Tetrad** A group of four cocci.

■ **Tetrapod** A vertebrate animal with four limbs.

■ **Texas fever** The causal agent is *Babesia bigemina*. It is a typical babesia. The disease is essentially a peracute anaemia.

■ **Texture** The structure or constitution of tissue.

■ **Thalami** These are two oval structures of grey matter placed at the top of the midbrain.

■ **Thalamus** (in anatomy) Part of vertebrate forebrain that lies above the hypothalamus and relays sensory nerve impulses.

■ **Theileria** Protozoan infection caused by *T. annulata*. Symptom–High fever.

■ **Theileriosis** Infection with tick-borne parasites of the *Theileridae*.

■ **Thelazia** Eye worms.

■ **Theory** The doctrine or the principles underlying an art as distinguished from the practice of that particular art.

■ **Therapeutics** The science and art of healing.

■ **Therapy** The treatment of disease; therapeutics.

■ **Therm(o)** Heat.

■ **Thermoduric** bacteria Organisms which grow optimally at temperatures from 120–160°F (50–60°C) and are able to survive temperatures higher than 176°F (80°C), but lie dormant till favourable growth temperature is reached.

- **Thermolysis** Chemical dissociation by means of heat.

- **Therogenology** Study of animal reproduction.

- **Thiabendazole** A chemical which is used against parasitic worms. 13 species of gastro-intestinal roundworms in sheep are stated to be susceptible to the drug.

- **Thiamin or Thiamine** Thiamine hydrochloride, or vitamin B_1.

- **Third eye lid** or Nictitating mebrane It is a piece of thin T-shaped cartilage enveloped by a fold of conjunctiva. It is situated at the medial angle of the eye.

- **Thirst** Thirst is an increased desire for water.

- **Thoracic cavity / Thorax** It is a laterally compressed cone shaped cavity. The contents of the thoracic cavity are lungs, heart, thoracic part of esophagus and trachea.

- **Thoracic vertebrae** These vertebrae make the bony roof of the thoracic cavity along with the proximal ends of the ribs.

- **Thoracotomy** A surgical operation involving opening of the chest cavity.

- **Thorouhbred** The name of an English breed of racing horses.

- **Thread-worm** is a popular term for *oxyuris* worms.

- **Three day's sickness of cattle** also called Ephemeral fever, Dengue fever, is an acute, infectious, and transient fever accompanied by muscular pains, and lameness.

- **Three way cross** A system of breeding involving the mating of three different breeds used in rotation on crossbred females.

- **Threonine** One of the essential amino acids.

- **Thrombocytopenia** A reduction in the number of platelets in the blood.

- **Thrombosis** Isntravascular clotting of blood or clot formation in heart or blood vessel.

- **Thymine** A pyrimidine derivative and one of the major component bases of nucleotides and the nucleic acid DNA.

- **Thymus** An organ, present only in vertebrates, that is

concerned with development of lymphoid tissue.

■ **Thyroid gland** These are two triangular dark brown coloured glands situated at the ventrolateral aspect of the junction of larynx and trachea.

■ **Thyroxin** A hormone secreted by the thyroid gland.

■ **Tibia** The larger of the two bones of the lower hindlimb of terrestrial vertebrates. It articulates with the femur at the knee and with the tarsus at the ankle.

■ **Ticks** These are among the most serious parasites of domestic animals. They transmit numerous protozoal and viral diseaseas.

■ **Tincture** is an alcoholic solution, e.g. tincture of iodine.

■ **Titer** The quality of a substance required to react with or to correspond to a given amount of another substance.

■ **Tocopherol** Vitamin E.

■ **Tomography** The use of X-rays to photograph a selected plane of a human body with other planes eliminated.

■ **Tomy** is a suffix indicating an operation by cutting.

■ **Tongue** A muscular organ of vertebrates that in most species is attached to the floor of the mouth. It plays an important role in manipulating food during chewing and swallowing.

■ **Tonics** Class of drugs believed to be a panacea for any and all ills of an obscure nature. Tonics are most useful when given during the convalescent stages of debilitating diseases, fevers, and during recovery from starvation, exhaustion.

■ **Tonic spasms** Continuous spasms

■ **Tonsil** A mass of lymphoid tissue, several of which are situated at the back of the mouth and throat in higher vertebrates.

■ **Tonsillitis** Inflammation of the tonsils.

■ **Top cross** A cross in which superior or purebred individuals or breeds, usually males, are mated with inferior stock.

■ **Topical applications** of a drug are those made locally to the outside of the body.

■ **Topical** Pertaining to a particular area.

■ **Topographic** Anatomy Principal structures or organs of

any part of the body are described in relation to a definite and limited area of the surface.

■ **Torsion** Twisting, occasionally involves the intestine; pedicle of spleen, stomach, uterus, and spermatic cords.

■ **Torticolis** Twisting of neck with an unnatural position of the head.

■ **Total cell count** (standard plate count) The total number of bacteria or fungi both viable and non-viable in a sample of milk or dairy product.

■ **Total digestible nutrients** (TDN) A term in animal feeding which designates the sum of all the digestible organic nutrients.

■ **Total dry matter** Dry matter in feed is weight of feed minus water removed by oven drying.

■ **Touch** This sense depends upon receptors at the end of nerves, or upon the nerve endings themselves, impulses being transmitted to the outer layer of the brain spinal cord.

■ **Toxaemia** Toxaemia is the presence of toxins deriving from bacteria or produced by body cells in the bloodstream.

■ **Toxic** Of a poisonous nature.

■ **Toxicology** The science or study of poisons.

■ **Toxocara canis** A roundworm parasite of the dog and fox.

■ **Toxicology** It is a study of poisoning.

■ **Toxin** Any poisonous substance produced by a microorganism.

■ **Toxoplasmosis** Toxoplasmosis is a contagious disease of all species, including man caused by *Toxoplasma gondii*. Clinically it is manifested chiefly by abortion and stillbirths in ewes, by encephalitis, pneumonia and neonatal mortality.

■ **Trace mineral** Any one of several mineral elements that are required by animals in very minute amounts.

■ **Tracer element** A radioactive element used in biological and other research to trace the fate of a substance.

■ **Trachea** The windpipe in air-breathing vertebrates; a tube that conducts air from the throat to the bronchi.

■ **Tracheitis** Inflammation of the trachea.

■ **Tranquilizer** Drugs having sedative and anti-anxiety actions for use in anxiety neuroses.

■ **Trans** Across or beyond.

■ **Translocation** The attachment of a fragment of one chromosome to another which is not homologous to it.

■ **Trauma** Injury caused by sharp objects, blunt impact, falling etc.

■ **Traumatic** Reticul operitonitis Perforation of the wall of the reticulum by a sharp foreign body producing initially a local peritonitis.

■ **Trematoda** A class of parasitic flatworms comprising the flukes, such as *Fasciola* (Liver fluke).

■ **Tremors** Mild spasms and confined to group of muscles. Involuntary trembling.

■ **Trihybrid** An individual that is heterozygous for three different pairs of genes (alleles) such as AaBbCc.

■ **Troughs** Receptacles for water or feed.

■ **True albino** An individual with a white coat color and with pink eyes. Pigment is lacking in all external parts of the body.

■ **Tubal ligation** A surgical procedure that involves ligation (closure) of the fallopian tubes to prevent an unfertilized egg from reaching the uterus.

■ **Tuberculin** test A test for detection of past or present tuberculosis infection in an animal.

■ **Tuberculosis** The disease caused by *Mycobacterium bovis* is characterized by the progressive development of tubercles in any of the organs in most species.

■ **Tuboplasty** Reconstructive surgery on the fallopian tubes to correct abnormalities that cause infertility.

■ **Tumour** Synonym of neoplasm

■ **Tympanic mebrane** (eardrum) This is a thin membranous oval structure situated at the junction between the external acoustic meatus and tympanic cavity in a tilted manner.

■ **Tympany** See bloat.

■ **Typhilitis** Inflammation of the caecum or first part of the large intestine.

U/u

■ **U.S.P.** United States Pharmacopeia, a legally recognized compendium of standards for drugs, published by the United States Pharmacopeial Convention.

■ **Udder** See mammary gland.

■ **UHT (Ultra High Temperature)** UHT treatment is a technique for preserving milk and other liquid food products by exposing them to brief, intense heat to temperatures in the range of 135–140°C (275–285°F).

■ **Ulcer** Loss of entire epidermis and the base of ulcer lies in the subcutaneous tissue, submucosa or, even deeper.

■ **Ulcerative granuloma** Ulcerative granuloma is an infectious disease of pigs caused by the spirochaete, *Borrelia suilla*, characterized by the development of chronic ulcers on the skin and subcuatneous tissue.

■ **Ulna** The larger of the two bones, in the forearm of vertebrates.

■ **Ultrafiltration (UF)** A separation process using a membrane with extremely fine pores, only 1-20 nanometers (millionth of a millimeter) in diameter.

■ **Umbilical cord** The cord that connects the embryo to the placenta in mammals.

■ **Undecorticated crab meal** It is the undecomposed ground dried waste of the crab and contains the shell, viscera, and part or all of the flesh. It must contain not less than 25% protein.

■ **Uniparous animals / Monotonus** Which give birth to one youngone at one time.

■ **Unit** A specified measure of a physical quantity, such as length, mass, time, etc.

■ **Uperization** Sterilizing milk by direct injection of steam.

■ **Uraemia** A toxaemic syndrome in which there is retention of urea in the blood.

■ **Urea** White crystalline organic compound; the end product of protein and amino acid metabolism in animals. The principal nitrogen compound secreted in urine.

■ **Urease** An enzyme which acts on urea to produce carbon dioxide and ammonia.

■ **Ureter** These tubes, one for each kidney are formed in the renal pelvis and terminate by opening at the urinary bladder.

■ **Urethra** This tube extends from the neck of the bladder to the glans penis.

■ **Uric acid** The end product of purine breakdown in most –primates, birds, terrestrial reptiles, and insects.

■ **Urinary system** This system excretes waste products from blood. The organs of this system are kidneys, ureters, urinary bladder and urethra.

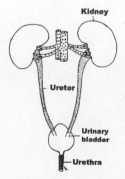

Kidney

Ureter

Urinary bladder

Urethra

URINARY SYSTEM

■ **Urination** or micturition Passing out of urine

■ **Urine** The aqueous fluid formed by the excretory organs of animals for the removal of metabolic waste prdoucts.

■ **Urolithiasis** Obstruction of the urethra by calculi characterized clinically by complete retention of urine and distension of the bladder.

■ **Uroliths** Urinary calculi

■ **U.S.P.** United States Pharmacopeia

■ **Ultra Sonography** the visualization of the deep structures of the body by recording the reflection of ultrasonic waves directed into the tissues.

■ **Ultra-violet rays** are used in the treatment of various skin diseases.

■ **Umbilicus** is another name for the navel.

■ **Unilateral** Affecting only one side.

■ **Ureter** The tubular organ through which urine passes from kidney to bladder.

■ **Uro** Urine

■ **Urticaria** See nettle Rash. Allergic reaction of skin characterized by pale, irregular elevated patches and severe itching.

■ **Uterine infections** These are discussed under uterus, diseases of and under infertility.

■ **U.S.P.** United States Pharmacopeia, a legally recognized compendium of standards for drugs, published by the United States Pharmacopeial Convention.

■ **Uterus** The portion of the reproductive tract in which the foetus develops. It is made up of two horns which lead into fallopian tubes.

❑

■ **Vaccination** A practice of artificially building up body immunity against specific infectious disease through inoculation with a specific antigen.

■ **Vaccine** Biological agent or an antigen (substances from organisms) which consists of a live, non-virulent or attenuated or dead bacterium or virus and is administered to produce or artificially increase immunity to a particular disease.

■ **Vacreation** Pasteurization of milk/cream under reduced pressure by direct steam.

■ **Vagina** It is a muscular tube extends from cervix to vulva.

■ **Vaginitis** Inflammation of the vaginal mucosa.

■ **Valvular Disease** Disease of the heart valves interferes with the normal flow of blood through the cardiac orifices.

■ **Vanaspati** Hydrogenated oils of vegetable origin (resembling ghee).

■ **Vancomycin** An antibiotic that inhibits cell wall synthesis.

■ **Vanadium** Element which is not shown to be essential but found in several animal tissues, and believed to play a biological role.

■ **Variance** A statistical term which indicates the amount of variation within a population. It is equal to the squared deviations from the mean (summed).

■ **Vas deferens** (ductus deferens, spermatic duct etc) The tube leading from the tail of the epididymus to the urethra.

■ **Vas efferens** Vessels that convey fluid away from a structure or part.

■ **Vasoconstriction** The reduction in the internal diameter of blood vessels, especially arteriole; or capillaries.

■ **Vasoconstrictor** Any agent which causes a narrowing of the lumen of blood vessels.

■ **Vasoconstrictor drugs** Refers to the drugs that are able to reduce the calibre of blood vessels, especially arterioles, by producing contraction of their smoother muscle.

■ **Vasodilation (vasodilatation)** The increase in the internal diameter of blood vessels, especially arterioles or capillaries.

■ **Vasodilator** Any agent which causes a widening of the lumen of blood vessels.

■ **Vector** In biology, any agent, but usually an insect, which is a carrier of a disease producing microorganism which it transmits from animal or plant to another, thus spreading disease.

■ **VEF** Viable embryo per flush.

■ **Vegetable drugs** The roots, leaves, and barks of plants used in the treatment of disease.

■ **Vegetable toned milk** Milk protein of skim milk powder is substituted by vegetable protein isolated from groundnut.

■ **Vehicles** Vehicles or solvents are used to solubilize drugs to render them more palatable.

■ **Veins** The systemic veins drain blood different tissues of the body to the heart.

■ **Venom** Poison or toxic substance secreted by insect or serpent.

■ **Vagotomy** Severing of the vagus nerve.

■ **Vancomycin** An antibiotic produced by Streptomytes or Orientals.

■ **Vas (o)** Vessel; duct.

■ **Vasectomised** A male animal in which the *vas deferens* has been cut.

■ **Vasopressin** A hormone secreted by the posterior lobe of the pituitary gland.

■ **Vegetable** Pertaining to or derived from plants.

■ **Venereal diseases** Two human venereal diseases—syphilis and gonorrhoea.

■ **Vent** Opening of cloaca in birds.

■ **Ventilation** Act of supplying a room continuously with fresh air.

■ **Ventral** Pertaining to the abdomen.

■ **Ventral/Inferior** Directed downwards towards grounds.

■ **Vermicide** A substance which kills worms.

■ **Vertebra** Any of the bones that make up the vertebral column.

■ **Vertebral column** (backbone; spinal column; spine) A flexible bony column in vertebrates that extends down the long axis of the body and provides the main skeletal support.

■ **Vertebrata (Craniata)** The largest subphylum of the Chordata.

■ **Vesicles/bullae** Circumscribed elevations produced by accumulation of fluid in or immediately beneath the epidermis.

■ **Vesicular exanthema** Vesicular exanthema is an acute, febrile, infectious disease of swine caused by a virus.

■ **Vesicular stomatitis** Vesicular stomatitis is an infectious disease caused by a virus and characterized clinically by the development of vesicles in the mouth and on the feet.

■ **Vestibule** It is a bony cavity placed medial to the tympanic cavity *or* The portion of the female reproductive tract lying just inside the vulvar opening and extending back to a point just beyond the opening to the urethra.

■ **Vestigial organ** Any part of an organism that has diminished in size during its evolution.

■ **Veterinary Bacteriology** It includes those microorganisms which affect the health of animals only.

■ **VFA** (Volatile fatty acids) Commonly used in reference to acetic, propionic, and butyric acids produced in the digestive tract.

■ **Vibrio** A curved or comma-shaped bacterium which is Gram-negative, motile and facultatively anaerobe.

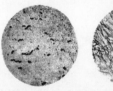

VIBRIO FETUS

■ **Villi** Small thread-like projectins attached to the interior side of the wall of the small intestine.

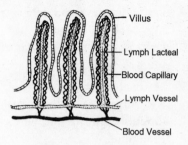

- Villus
- Lymph Lacteal
- Blood Capillary
- Lymph Vessel
- Blood Vessel

VILLI OF INTESTINE

■ **Viroid** Name given to a particle of nucleic acid which is much smaller than a virus but lacks the tough protein coat of the virus.

■ **Virology** The study of the filterable viruses which affect man and animals.

■ **Virucide** Which kills a virus is a virucide.

■ **Virulence** Infectiousness, the disease producing power of a microorganism.

■ **Virus** The smallest type of micro-organism, cannot reproduce outside a living cell. Cause of most major diseases.

■ **Viscera** The organs of the great cavities of the body which are normally removed upon slaughter.

■ **Vitamins** Organic feed substances necessary in small amounts for normal metabolism of the animal.

■ **Vitreous body** A poorly set jelly like substance occupies the posterior compartment of the eye ball.

■ **Viviparous** Producing living young by true birth, as an mammals.

■ **Volatile oils** Volatile oils are volatilized by heat, also called essential oils.

■ **Volvulus** Twisting of bowel on long axis of mesentery resulting obstruction.

■ **Vomiting** A mechanism usually protective and reverse to peristaltic movement with the function of removing excessive quantities of ingesta or toxic material from stomach.

■ **Vulva** The external opening of the female reproductive (and urogenital) tract.

■ **Vulvitis** Inflammation of the vulva.

■ **Vulvovaginitis** Inflammation of the vulva and vagina.

■ **Vagotomy** Severing of the vagus nerve.

■ **Ventricle** is the term applied to the two larger cavities of the heart.

■ **Vertigo** Chronic asthma accompanied by a weak heart, turning giddy and falling after severe attack of coughing.

■ **Vesicles, Seminal** These secondary sex glands, like the prosate, have openings into the urethra and are situated close to the neck of the urinary bladder.

■ **Veterinary** Pertaining to domestic animals and their diseases.

■ **Veterinary profession** This comprises those engaged in private practice, in the Animal Health Division of the Ministry of Agriculture, the Royal Army Veterinary Corps, overseas veterinary services, in research and teaching at the universities at ARC research establishments in AI Centres.

■ **Vial** Ampoule or a small bottle.

■ **Vibrio foetus** Organism causing abortion.

■ **Vices** or **Viciousness** Definition comprehensive enough to include 'bad habits'.

■ **Viral** Relating to viruses.

■ **Viral infections** caused by virus and cannot be controlled by antibiotics.

■ **Virginiamycin** An antibiotic which may be included in live-stock rations.

■ **Virologist** A microbiologist specializing in virology.

■ **Virucidal** Capable of neutralizing or destroying a virus.

■ **Vision** The capacity for being able to appreciate the position of objects in the outside world.

■ **Voice** is the sound produced as the result of the vibration of a column of air forced through the larynx by contraction of the respiratory muscles.

■ **Volar** At the back of the fore-limb.

■ **Voluntary** Accomplished in accordance with the wall.

❏

Wallerian degeneration Swelling and degeneration of both axon and myelin-sheath.

W.H.O. World Health Organization, an international agency associates with the United Nations in based in Geneva.

Warbles are swellings about the size of a marble or small walnut occurring upon the backs of cattle in spring and early summer caused by maggot of one of the warble flies.

WARBLES

MAGGOTS

Warts are small solid growths arising upon the surface of the skin or mucous membrane in all the domestic animals.

Water Clear, colorless, odorless, tasteless liquid, H_2O.

Water-borne Spread or transmitted by drinking water.

Watt A unit of electric power.

Wax A plastic substance deposited by insects or obtained from plants.

Weals are raised white areas of the skin which possess reddened margins. They may result from sharp blows or from continued pressure against some hard object.

Weaving is a habit of horses —swinging the head and neck and the anterior parts of the body backwards and forwards, so that the weights rest alternately upon each fore-limb.

Weaning To accustom young calves to take feed otherwise than by suckling.

Weight Heaviness; the degree to which a body is drawn toward the earth by gravity.

Wetting agents Wetting agents–usually sulphonated alcohols–may be added to detergents to improve their effectiveness.

■ **Wheat middlings** Consists of fine particles of wheat bran, wheat shorts (a by-product of milling that consists of bran, germ and coarse meal) and some of the offal from the 'tail of the mill'.

■ **Wheel** See Urticaria.

■ **Wheezing** Sound produced due to stenosis of the nasal passages.

■ **Whelping** parturition, in the bitch.

■ **Whey** The watery part which is separated from the curd after milk is coagulated for cheese making.

■ **Whipworm** is the popular name for the *Trichuris* found in caecum.

■ **Whistling** is a defect affecting the respiratory system of the horse. It is similar to roaring, but the not emitted is higher pitched.

■ **White muscle disease** is another name for the result of Vitamin E deficiency.

■ **White matter** It is remaining below the grey matter and composed of three groups of medullated fibers.

■ **White scour** is a contagious bacterial disease affecting calves within the first 3 weeks of life in which the chief symptoms are severe whitish diarrohea, emaciation and weakness. *Cause* is usually *E.Coli, Proteus vulgaris* and *Pseudomonas pyocyanea.*

■ **White spotted kidney** Focal interstitial nephritis.

■ **Whole blood** Whole blood is used primarily for immediate transfusion because it cannot be stored indefinitely.

■ **Whole milk powder** When water is removed from milk, dried whole milk is the result.

■ **Whorl** A swirl, or cowlick, in the hair coat of an animal.

■ **Winter dysentery of cattle** Winter dysentery is a highly contagious disease of cattle characterized by a brief attack of severe diarrhoea and sometimes dysentery caused by vibrio spp.

■ **Withers** The highest part of the back immediately behind where the neck joins it, formed by the first few thoracic vertebrae.

■ **Windpipe** the trachea.

■ **Winking** Quick opening and closing of the eyelids.

■ **Wire** A slender, elongated, flexible structure of metal.

■ **Womb** See uterus.

■ **Wooden tongue** or **Woody tongue** Actinobacillosis.

■ **Worms** Parasitic worms include round worms, tapeworms, and flukes.

■ **Wounds** A wound may be defined as a breach of the continuity of the tissues of the body produced by violence.

❑

■ **Xanthine** An intermediate in the metabolism of purines; related to uric acid.

■ **Xeroderma** Dryness of the skin.

■ **Xerophthalmia** Dry infected eye condition caused by lack of vitamin A.

■ **X-rays** Electromagnetic radiation of shorter wavelength than ultraviolet radiation and longer wavelength than gamma radiation.

■ **Xylose** A 5 carbon aldehyde sugar that is not metabolised by the body.

■ **Xenoparasite** Organism not usually parasitic on a particular species, but which becomes so because of a weakened condition of the host.

■ **Xero** Dry; dryness.

■ **Xiphoid** Sword-shaped.

❏

Y/y

■ **Yak** A wild or domesticated species of ox (*Bos grunniens*) of the high plateaus and mountains of Tibet and Central Asia, covered with a thick coat of long silky hair, that of the lower parts hanging down almost to the ground.

■ **Yeasts** Yeasts are generally characterized by their morphology and their reproduction by budding.

■ **Yield** To produce or give forth. In relation to dairy, milk produced by an animal per day.

■ **Yoghurt** A fermented, slightly acid semi-fluid milk product made of skimmed milk and milk solids to which culture of two bacteria (*Lactobacillus bulgaricus and Streptococcus thermophilus*) are added . Yoghurt is considered to repress undesired bacteria in the bowels.

■ **Yolk** The food stored in an egg for the use of the embryo.

■ **Yolk sac** It is very small sac which provides nutrition to the embryo.

■ **Yawn** A deep, involuntary inspiration with the mouth open.

■ **Yeast** is a valuable source of Vitamin B.

■ **Yelt** A female pig intended for breeding.

■ **Yolk** the stored nutrient of the ovum.

❑

■ **Zein** A protein of low biological value present in maize, deficient in lysine and tryptophan.

■ **Zinc bacitracin** Productivity promoter.

■ **Zona pellucida** A translucent, elastic, noncellular layer surrounding the ovum of many mammals.

■ **Zoology** The scientific study of animals, including their anatomy, physiology, biochemistry, genetics, ecology, evolution, and behaviour.

■ **Zoonosis** Any disease communicable from one animal to another and or to man.

■ **Zurpi** The name given to sun-dried butter-milk in Nepal and known as 'kurud' in Afghanistan.

■ **Zygote** The original cell formed by the fusion of the sperm and ovum which possesses all the hereditary characteristics that will develop in the new individual and many of those possessed by the race from which it comes.

■ **Zinc** Chemical element, its salts are often poisonous.

■ **Zone** An encircling region or area, by extension, any area with specific characteristics.

■ **Zoo pathology** The science of the diseases of animals.

■ **Zoo therapeutics** Veterinary medicine.

■ **Zoogamous** Acquired from animals.

■ **Zoophilia** Abnormal fondness for animals.

■ **Zoophobia** Abnormal fear of animals.

■ **Zoophyte** Any plantlike animal.

■ **Zoospore** A motile reproductive spore.

■ **Zootechny** Animal management.

■ **Zootomy** The dissection or anatomy of animals.

■ **Zygote intra-fallopian transfer** In vitro fertilization with a transfer of the zygote into the fallopian tube.

■ **Zymogen** The inactive form of an enzyme.

❏

Lotus Illustrated Dictionaries for Rs. 95 each

Agriculture

Anthropology

Architeture

Archaeology

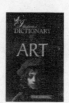
Art

Astronomy

Banking
Finance
& Accounting

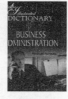
Business
Administration

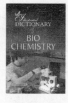
Bio Chemistry

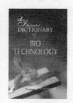
Bio
Technology

Biology

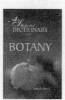
Botany

Chemical
Engineering

Chemistry

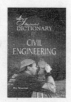
Civil
Engineering

Computer
Science

Commerce

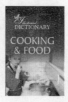
Cooking &
Food

Culture

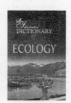
Ecology

Lotus Illustrated Dictionaries for Rs. 95 each

| Economics | Education | Electrical Engineering | Electronics & Telecommunication | Environmental Studies |

| Festival | Geography | Geology | Genetic Engineering | Health Nutrition |

   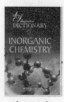

| History | Internet | IT | Inorganic Chemistry | Law |

  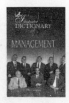 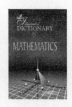

| Library & Information Science | Literature | Management | Mathematics | Managment |

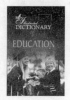
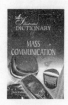 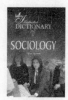
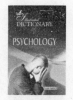 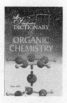 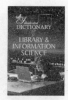 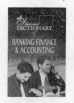
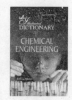 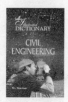   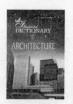
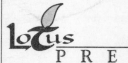